Treatment Plans and Interventions for Bulimia and Binge–Eating Disorder

Rene D. Zweig
Robert L. Leahy

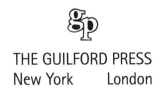

THE GUILFORD PRESS
New York   London

© 2012 The Guilford Press
A Division of Guilford Publications, Inc.
72 Spring Street, New York, NY 10012
www.guilford.com

Printed in the United States of America

This book is printed on acid-free paper.

Last digit is print number: 9   8   7   6   5   4   3   2   1

The authors have checked with sources believed to be reliable in their efforts to provide information that is complete and generally in accord with the standards of practice that are accepted at the time of publication. However, in view of the possibility of human error or changes in behavioral, mental health, or medical sciences, neither the authors, nor the editor and publisher, nor any other party who has been involved in the preparation or publication of this work warrants that the information contained herein is in every respect accurate or complete, and they are not responsible for any errors or omissions or the results obtained from the use of such information. Readers are encouraged to confirm the information contained in this book with other sources.

Library of Congress Cataloging-in-Publication data is available from the publisher.

ISBN 978-1-4625-0258-5

TREATMENT PLANS AND INTERVENTIONS FOR BULIMIA AND BINGE-EATING DISORDER

TREATMENT PLANS AND INTERVENTIONS
FOR EVIDENCE–BASED PSYCHOTHERAPY

Robert L. Leahy, Series Editor

This series provides psychotherapy practitioners with a wealth of practical tools for treating clients with a range of presenting problems. Each volume synthesizes current information on a particular disorder or clinical population; demonstrates how to develop specific, tailored treatment plans; and describes interventions proven to reduce distress and alleviate symptoms. Step-by-step guidelines for planning and implementing treatment are illustrated with rich case examples. User-friendly features include reproducible self-report forms, handouts, and symptom checklists, all in a convenient large-size format. Specific strategies for handling treatment roadblocks are also detailed. Emphasizing a collaborative approach to treatment, books in this series enable therapists to offer their clients the very best in evidence-based practice.

TREATMENT PLANS AND INTERVENTIONS FOR DEPRESSION
AND ANXIETY DISORDERS, SECOND EDITION
Robert L. Leahy, Stephen J. F. Holland, and Lata K. McGinn

TREATMENT PLANS AND INTERVENTIONS FOR BULIMIA
AND BINGE-EATING DISORDER
Rene D. Zweig and Robert L. Leahy

For Matt and Ethan
—R. D. Z.

For Helen
—R. L. L.

About the Authors

Rene D. Zweig, PhD, is Director of Union Square Cognitive Therapy, a full-time private practice in New York City. Previously, she directed the Eating Disorders and Weight Management Program at the American Institute for Cognitive Therapy. Dr. Zweig is Adjunct Clinical Supervisor at the Ferkauf Graduate School of Psychology at Yeshiva University and a Diplomate of the Academy of Cognitive Therapy.

Robert L. Leahy, PhD, is Director of the American Institute for Cognitive Therapy in New York City and Clinical Professor of Psychology in the Department of Psychiatry at Weill Cornell Medical College. He is the author or editor of 19 books on cognitive therapy and psychological processes, including the professional books *Cognitive Therapy Techniques* and *Overcoming Resistance in Cognitive Therapy* and the popular books *The Worry Cure* and *Beat the Blues Before They Beat You.* Dr. Leahy is Past President of the Association for Behavioral and Cognitive Therapies, the International Association for Cognitive Psychotherapy, and the Academy of Cognitive Therapy. He is a recipient of the Aaron T. Beck Award for Sustained and Enduring Contributions to Cognitive Therapy. He has given workshops worldwide and has appeared frequently in the popular media.

Contents

List of Figures, Tables, and Forms

FIGURES

TABLES

FORMS

CHAPTER 1

Introduction

Approximately 5 million Americans meet diagnostic criteria for an eating disorder every year (Becker, Grinspoon, Klibanski, & Herzog, 1999; Hudson, Hiripi, Pope, & Kessler, 2007). The eating disorders, which include bulimia nervosa (BN), anorexia nervosa (AN), and eating disorder not otherwise specified (EDNOS), are all serious psychological disorders.* The purpose of this book is to provide therapists and other health care practitioners with a comprehensive treatment model and empirically supported interventions for BN. Information is also provided to allow practitioners to adapt this treatment for patients with EDNOS, including binge-eating disorder (BED), purging disorder, and subthreshold BN.

Although eating disorders are relatively uncommon psychiatric illnesses, they warrant careful study and efficacious treatment because of their chronic, severe nature. Lifetime prevalence estimates of AN, BN, and BED are 0.9%, 1.5%, and 3.5% among women, respectively, and 0.3%, 0.5%, and 2.0% among men, respectively (Hudson et al., 2007). Individuals may meet diagnostic criteria for more than one eating disorder over their lifetime, and relapse following treatment is not uncommon. Regardless of the specific diagnosis, individuals with an eating disorder are more likely than those without an eating disorder to have a comorbid Axis I diagnosis, particularly major depression, obsessive–compulsive disorder, or a substance use disorder (Kaye, Bulik, et al., 2004). Suicidality, poor body image, perfectionism, and low self-image also commonly co-occur with BN (Fink, Smith, Gordon, Holm-Denoma, & Joiner, 2009; Wade, 2007). Like the other eating disorders, BN is associated with an elevated mortality risk, health complications, dental erosion, disrupted interpersonal relationships, and impairment in educational/employment pursuits. Effective treatment can reverse the course of BN and improve the patient's functioning across all domains. Without treatment, BN, like all the eating disorders, is chronic (Fairburn, Cooper, Doll, Norman, & O'Connor, 2000).

BN was first described as a distinct disorder in 1979 (Russell, 1979). Since that time, a significant amount of progress has been made in understanding BN and in developing effective treatments (Mitchell, Agras, & Wonderlich, 2007; Steinhausen & Weber, 2009). BN is more common than once thought, afflicting approximately 1.5% of women and 0.5% of men in their

---

*The *Diagnostic and Statistical Manual of Mental Disorders* (DSM-IV-TR; American Psychiatric Association, 2000) recognizes anorexia nervosa, bulimia nervosa, and eating disorder not otherwise specified as distinct disorders, and also lists binge-eating disorder separately as a provisional disorder requiring further study (see Table 1.1).

TABLE 1.1. Diagnostic Criteria for the Eating Disorders

	Bulimia nervosa	Anorexia nervosa	Eating disorder not otherwise specified
DSM-IV-TR diagnostic code	307.51	307.1	307.50
Prevalence	Females, 1.5% lifetime Males, 0.5% lifetime	Females, 0.9% lifetime Males, 0.3% lifetime	For BED: Females, 3.5% Males, 2.0%
Symptoms	1. At least twice-weekly episodes of binge eating that include loss of control and consumption of an objectively large quantity of food during a 2-hour period. 2. Use of compensatory behaviors at least twice weekly to avoid weight gain. 3. Bingeing and purging has occurred for at least 3 months. 4. Self-worth largely determined by perceived shape/weight.	1. Body weight below 85% of expected normal for age and height. 2. Extreme fear of weight gain. 3. Distorted body image, self-worth based largely on body weight, and minimizing of the seriousness of low body weight. 4. Amenorrhea.	Disorders of eating that are clinically significant, cause distress, and/or impair functioning that do not meet the criteria for AN or BN. May include BED, purging disorder, mixed eating disorder symptoms, subthreshhold BN, and subthreshhold AN.

Note. Data from American Psychiatric Association (2000) and Hudson, Hiripi, Pope, and Kessler (2007).

lifetimes (Hudson et al., 2007). In addition to its direct effect on health, BN often negatively affects work, school, social, and familial responsibilities (Hudson et al., 2007). Patients with BN also have elevated rates of suicide attempts, self-injurious behavior, major depression and other Axis I disorders, Axis II disorders, and substance abuse. Purging and other symptoms of BN can cause irreversible dental and medical consequences. Despite the severity of the disorder and the availability of efficacious psychological treatments, most patients with BN remain undertreated (Wells & Sadowski, 2001). Fewer than 50% of patients with BN seek treatment specifically for their eating disorder, and physicians typically do not screen their patients for symptoms of BN (Hudson et al., 2007).

Although this book focuses primarily on the cognitive-behavioral treatment of BN, there is considerable overlap in both the symptoms and treatment of all the eating disorders. AN, BN, and EDNOS, which includes subthreshold eating disorders, BED, and purging disorder, are recognized as separate disorders in the American Psychiatric Association's current diagnostic manual.* Yet all the eating disorders share several common core features: a preoccupation with shape, weight, and food intake; a strong desire to be thin; use of extreme measures to try to achieve a desirable shape; distorted body image; unrealistic expectations about body shape and composition; perfectionism; discomfort eating in the presence of others; and a lack of healthy emotional coping skills. Additional information about the current diagnostic system and the "transdiagnosis" of eating disorders can be found in Appendix A. In recognition of the overlap in symptoms across eating disorder diagnoses, this book provides information for clinicians to adapt treatment for patients with BED, purging disorder, subthreshold BN, and other variations of EDNOS.

RATIONALE FOR COGNITIVE–BEHAVIORAL TREATMENT

BN was first recognized by the DSM in 1980, and effective psychological treatments have since been developed. Of all the psychological treatments in use for the eating disorders, cognitive-behavioral therapy (CBT) is considered to be most efficacious for BN (Fairburn & Harrison, 2003; Wilson & Fairburn, 2002). Interpersonal psychotherapy (IPT) may be as effective as CBT in the treatment of BN, although patients treated with IPT recovered significantly more slowly than with those treated with CBT (Agras, Walsh, Fairburn, Wilson, & Kraemer, 2000). IPT is a manualized, short-term, nondirective treatment that was originally developed for depression and has since been adapted to treat BN. IPT treatment sessions focus on identifying and changing the maladaptive interpersonal context in which the eating disorder developed and is maintained, and the eating disorder is not discussed directly in these sessions. Some early evidence supports the use of dialectical behavior therapy (DBT) for the treatment of BN (Safer, Telch, & Agras, 2001). DBT has been used as a stand-alone treatment for BN and also in conjunction with CBT protocols. DBT effectively targets the link between binge eating and negative affect by teaching patients emotion regulation skills. Additional research is needed, however, to determine whether DBT is as effective as CBT in the treatment of BN or whether it is particularly useful with a specific subset of patients.

CBT for BN was given an "A" evidence grade by the United Kingdom's National Institute for Clinical Excellence (2004) guidelines, which indicates that CBT is an evidence-based treatment supported by multiple randomized control trials. Nearly half of patients make a full recovery after receiving CBT for BN, and many more experience a significant reduction in their bingeing, purging, and dietary restriction (Agras, Walsh, et al., 2000). Following treatment, a significant proportion of patients remain in full or partial remission (Fairburn et al., 1995; Keel, Mitchell, Miller, Davis, & Crow, 1999).

Eating disorders have been incorrectly described as an exaggerated form of body dissatis-

---

*As a result of recognized problems with the current diagnostic criteria for eating disorders, including the elevated prevalence of EDNOS diagnoses, several changes to the diagnostic criteria have been proposed by the Eating Disorders Work Group that are likely to be included the next revision of the *Diagnostic and Statistical Manual of Mental Disorders* (DSM-5; Eating Disorders Work Group, American Psychiatric Association, 2010). DSM-5 is due to be published in May 2013. The proposed changes for DSM-5 include recognizing BED as a distinct diagnostic category no longer subsumed under EDNOS, removing amenorrhea from the diagnostic criteria for AN, and delineating several conditions that will fall under the EDNOS diagnostic category: atypical AN; subthreshold BN; subthreshold BED; purging disorder; night-eating syndrome; and other feeding or eating condition not otherwise classified.

faction. Among females in America, Europe, and many other areas, body dissatisfaction is so prevalent that it has been coined "normative discontent" (Rodin, Silberstein, & Striegel-Moore, 1984). Body image dissatisfaction and thin weight ideals are more common in women from wealthier nations and in the Americas than other areas of the world (Swami et al., 2010). More than one-half of American women of all ages report feeling dissatisfied with their bodies (Cash & Henry, 1995; Frederick, Peplau, & Lever, 2006). This dissatisfaction is typically focused on one's body weight, the shape of the lower body, and the shape of the torso (waist). However, normative discontent is substantially different from and is not synonymous with eating disorder symptomatology. Individuals can dislike aspects of their bodies without engaging in extreme measures to maintain thinness, without threatening their physical and mental well-being, without basing their self-worth on body weight alone, and without interfering with their daily functioning. Eating disorders, in contrast, are chronic, are severe, and do warrant evidence-based intervention.

LEVEL-OF-CARE DECISION MAKING

Although this book focuses on cognitive-behavioral treatment for eating disorders in individual and outpatient settings, treatment is available in multiple settings with varying intensities. Treatment for BN can occur in outpatient, intensive outpatient, inpatient, or long-term residential settings. Treatment may take place in a medical center, psychiatric hospital, community clinic, specialty clinic, or private practice. Treatment can be provided by any qualified professional, including, but not limited to, psychologists, psychiatrists, social workers, mental health counselors, nutritionists, internists, and nurse practitioners (hereafter referred to as "the therapist"). The therapist may utilize individual sessions, group therapy, guided self-help, teleconferencing or videoconferencing, or any combination of these. Severity of presenting symptoms, duration of illness, comorbidity, and availability of treatment are all factors that may affect the setting in which treatment is provided.

The American Psychiatric Association (2006) recommends a stepped-care model to determine the appropriate level of treatment, meaning that the lowest reasonable level of treatment should first be utilized with any given patient. From there, the level of care can be stepped up (or down) as necessary. This approach has the advantage of balancing the least disruptive level of care with one that is maximally effective for the patient. The stepped-care model means that the majority of patients, including those with severe symptoms and a long eating disorder history, can receive cognitive-behavioral treatment in an outpatient setting. In fact, intensive outpatient and inpatient treatments, although more time intensive and costly, are not automatically more effective than outpatient cognitive-behavioral treatment (Meads, Gold, & Burls, 2001). Most patients with BN are treated in an outpatient setting, with only 13% receiving hospitalization (Striegel-Moore, Leslie, Petrill, Garvin, & Rosenheck, 2000). A subset of patients with BN remit without formal treatment, either on their own or by using a self-help workbook (Carter et al., 2003).

Treatment decisions are best made after a comprehensive psychological and medical assessment of the patient (see Appendix B). This assessment may include the patient's presenting symptoms, body weight, current food intake, frequency of purging behaviors, vital signs, electrolyte levels, concurrent medical consequences, psychiatric comorbidity, past or present suicidality, past treatment episodes, ability to meet daily responsibilities, and motivation for treatment. In addition, practical concerns such as availability of and proximity to treatment as well as health insurance coverage may factor into level-of-care decisions.

In instances where medical or psychological stabilization is required, inpatient treatment should be recommended to patients. Hospitalization is more common among patients with AN than those with BN or EDNOS, but it may be warranted in severe forms of these eating disorders. The *Practice Guideline for the Treatment of Patients with Eating Disorders* (American Psychiatric Association, 2006) suggests several circumstances under which inpatient treatment or medical hospitalization should be considered by the therapist and recommended to patients (see Table 1.2). A body mass index (BMI) below 18.5 is considered underweight and is a defining symptom of AN. Patients are often immediately hospitalized if their BMI is below 18.0 because this index suggests the need for medical stabilization and monitored refeeding. BMI is a standardized reference for body weight that takes height into account, and it is most often used to categorize patients as underweight, normal weight, or overweight (see Appendix B for more information). No single criterion mandates inpatient treatment, although an immediate referral is warranted if there is any symptom that represents imminent harm to patients (e.g., suicidality, dangerously low body weight, refusal to eat, electrolyte abnormalities). In that case, a referral should be made to an inpatient treatment setting that can provide constant supervision and/or refeeding. In addition, lack of progress in outpatient or intensive outpatient treatment or the intensification of symptoms while in a lower level of care also suggests the need for a more structured, more intensive treatment environment.

Intensive outpatient treatment is often utilized as an alternative to weekly outpatient treat-

---

TABLE 1.2. Circumstances That Warrant Inpatient Hospitalization

Hospitalization should be considered when the patient displays any one or more of the following symptoms:

- Below 85% of expected body weight *or* BMI below 18.0.
- Severe resistance to and/or low motivation for change.
- Long duration of eating disorder.
- Purging multiple times daily.
- Lack of access to outpatient treatment.
- Low familial and social support for change.
- Amenorrhea.
- Acute or multiple comorbid psychiatric disorders.
- Concurrent alcohol or substance abuse.
- Strong risk or intent for suicide.
- Serious concurrent medical problems.
- Electrolyte imbalance.
- Abnormal vital signs such as pulse, blood pressure, or body temperature.
- Rapid rate of weight loss.

ment when more structure and stability would benefit the patient. This is often recommended when a patient is unemployed, severely depressed, or experiencing very chaotic eating and bingeing patterns. Intensive outpatient treatment typically includes a combination of individual and group therapy sessions held for several hours daily. The patient typically attends these programs for 3 or more days per week, either during the daytime or in the evenings. This level of treatment is often used as a step-down from successful inpatient treatment, although it also can be utilized as a first-line treatment or a step-up if a patient is not improving through outpatient treatment.

In the absence of severe psychiatric comorbidity or life-threatening medical consequences from the eating disorder, outpatient treatment can often be recommended as the first-line treatment. This treatment, described throughout this manual, can be provided through once- or twice-weekly individual psychotherapy sessions. At the outset of treatment, the therapist and patient can draft a treatment contract to stipulate that, although weekly outpatient treatment will first be utilized, the patient will be transferred to a higher level of care if substantial improvement is not made within 6 weeks. Treatment providers will then need to routinely assess which level of care and setting are appropriate for any given patient. Assessment is an ongoing process that should occur throughout treatment, not simply at the outset, because a patient may experience significant improvements, setbacks, or an onset of comorbid conditions that will affect the appropriate level of care.

Regardless of the level of care recommended, it is important that empirically supported treatments are utilized to maximize the potential for treatment response. For adults, CBT is widely considered to be the recommended first-line treatment for BN. For adolescents and children, both CBT and family-based treatment, also known as the Maudsley approach, have been shown to be efficacious (le Grange & Lock, 2009; Schmidt et al., 2007).

USING THIS TREATMENT PLANNER

This book is intended to be a comprehensive guide for clinicians who wish to provide CBT for BN. Included in this treatment planner are diagnostic criteria for the eating disorders, background information on the conceptualization and treatment of BN, assessment tools, a session-by-session protocol for the cognitive-behavioral treatment of BN, patient handouts and worksheets, and an extensive case example. Using these materials, the reader will be equipped to assess, diagnose, conceptualize, and treat a patient with BN. Suggestions are also provided for adapting this treatment for BED, purging disorder, subthreshold BN, and other variations of EDNOS. The included treatment planning materials are a synthesis of the original empirically supported treatment for BN, the transdiagnostic treatment for eating disorders, and current eating disorders treatment research (Fairburn et al., 2009; Fairburn, Marcus, & Wilson, 1993).

In this chapter we have discussed the symptoms of eating disorders, their diagnosis, treatment outcome research, common comorbid psychopathology, and level-of-care decision making as well as basic information about CBT and its application to BN. In Chapter 2 we go into more detail about BN and offer a cognitive-behavioral model for understanding it. From there, we provide descriptions of the common comorbid medical and psychiatric problems as well as information about the efficacy of psychotropic medications most often prescribed for BN. Collaboration with a full treatment team, including an internist, a psychiatrist, and a nutritionist, is strongly encouraged.

Chapter 3 consists of detailed information to assist any therapist with assessment and case conceptualization of a patient with an eating disorder.

The treatment plan is included in Chapter 4. We present session-by-session suggestions for the treatment of BN, including thorough descriptions of interventions, in-session worksheets, patient handouts, and suggestions for between-session homework. This 20-session treatment plan is appropriate for adult and adolescent patients seeking outpatient treatment for BN, and it can be readily adapted for patients with EDNOS. A section on handling "roadblocks" and managing treatment resistance is provided at the end of Chapter 4 to assist the therapist with effective treatment implementation.

To illustrate the treatment plan in action, Chapter 5 offers a case example that parallels the session-by-session treatment planner. For each of the patient worksheets suggested in Chapter 4, a completed sample is shown with the case example in Chapter 5. Before providing this treatment, the therapist should become familiar with the entire treatment protocol. In addition, consistent with the ethical guidelines for clinical conduct, clinical supervision should be sought prior to treating an individual when the presenting problems are outside the bounds of the therapist's expertise.

Many patients presenting for treatment for BN will be utilizing their health insurance to cover or offset the cost of treatment. In this era of managed health care, the patient's health care provider often requires the therapist to provide initial diagnostic reports, updates on treatment progress, and requests for additional sessions in order to cover the patient's treatment costs. Chapter 6 discusses how to communicate effectively with the managed care organization. This chapter includes information on eating disorder diagnoses, a sample treatment report, lists of symptoms and interventions to be included in treatment reports, and guidelines for requesting additional sessions.

Appendix A provides additional information about the transdiagnostic theory and updated research on the eating disorders. Appendix B includes several assessment instruments that will help clinicians conduct proper evaluations at intake and throughout treatment. Appendix C offers suggestions for background reading in CBT for those clinicians who wish to better understand this treatment modality. Patients and their families often benefit from reading as an adjunct to their treatment, both for psychoeducation and to reinforce concepts discussed in treatment sessions; suggested reading materials for patients and their families also are provided in Appendix C.

Experienced clinicians, new professionals, and graduate students should all find useful information within this planner to guide their treatment of eating disorders. Although no prior training in CBT is required for use of this treatment planner, a basic knowledge of the key concepts will be useful for any practitioner.

The confines of this treatment planner are as important to mention as its contents. The cognitive-behavioral interventions are intended to be a stand-alone treatment for adults and adolescents with BN, and not to be used piecemeal or in an adjunctive manner. Instead, this treatment has been shown to be effective when its interventions are utilized all together and as part of a cognitive-behavioral case conceptualization (see Chapter 3). Although the treatment interventions should be utilized largely as described, we expect you will adapt treatment to fit each patient's unique symptom and cognitive profile. Likewise, the interventions described herein can be adapted for use with patients with subthreshold BN and with EDNOS. CBT for BED, for example, is quite similar to the treatment described in Chapter 4, although there is no need to focus on purging. This treatment plan also may be adapted for adolescents with BN. The current research literature suggests that family-based treatment is most effective for adolescents with AN, although results are less clear for adolescents with BN (Eisler et al., 1997; le Grange, Crosby, Rathouz, & Leventhal, 2007). Either CBT or family-based treatment may be efficacious for adolescents with BN (Schmidt et al., 2007).

Although this treatment planner may be useful for patients with various forms of an eating disorder, this treatment should not be utilized concurrently with weight reduction efforts. Dieting has been shown to exacerbate and maintain disordered eating regardless of diagnosis. Specifically, dietary restriction often precedes the onset of bingeing. Strict dietary rules, whether or not they are adhered to, are considered maintaining factors in BN, BED, and AN. Throughout this CBT for BN, there is an emphasis on reducing food rules and dietary restriction. Thus, active dieting is contraindicated for improvement in this treatment. Weight loss, where indicated, can be set as a treatment goal only once patients are abstinent from bingeing.

CHAPTER 2

Bulimia Nervosa

DESCRIPTION

Symptoms

BN consists of episodes of binge eating, purging or other compensatory behaviors following binges, and overevaluation of self based on body shape and weight (American Psychiatric Association, 2000). Binges are often, but not always, planned in advance. Between binge episodes, individuals with BN typically restrict their overall food intake and limit their choice of foods. Bingeing and purging symptoms must occur at least twice weekly for a period of 3 months to meet diagnostic criteria. Of the possible compensatory measures following binges, approximately 80–90% of patients with BN vomit, approximately 30% misuse laxatives, and others utilize fasting, excessive exercise, diuretics, enemas, and/or stimulants. BN may be subtyped as purging type (use of vomiting, laxatives, or diuretics) or nonpurging type (other compensatory measures, including fasting or exercise). Behaviors associated with BN typically occur in secret and, as with the other eating disorders, are characterized by rigidity, perfectionism, and strong reactions to negative mood states.

Prevalence and Life Course

The lifetime prevalence of BN is estimated at between 1 and 3% (American Psychiatric Association, 2000). Approximately 90% of patients with BN are female. BN typically arises during late adolescence or early adulthood, with a mean age of onset of 19.7 years (Hudson et al., 2007). BN can persist across the lifespan, and the mean duration of an episode is 8.3 years (Hudson et al., 2007). Without treatment, the natural course of BN is chronic (Fairburn et al., 2000). BN occurs in individuals of all body weights, although most individuals with BN are within a normal weight range. There is some indication that patients are likely to be overweight prior to onset of BN, and the onset of the disorder often arises after a period of restrictive dieting (Fairburn, Welch, Doll, Davies, & O'Connor, 1997; Patton, Selzer, Coffrey, Carlin, & Wolfe, 1999).

BN is associated with an elevated risk of mortality, and individuals with BN are more likely than their peers to attempt suicide (Keel & Mitchell, 1997; Pompili, Girardi, Tatarelli, Ruberto, & Tatarelli, 2006). Lifetime suicide attempts among patients with BN are estimated at between 11 and 40% (Franko et al., 2004; Pompili et al., 2006).

Genetic/Biological Factors

Research suggests that BN, like other eating disorders, has a strong genetic component (Kaye, Devlin, et al., 2004; Strober, Freeman, Lampert, Diamond, & Kaye, 2000). The rates of all eating disorders, including BN, are elevated in familial and twin studies of patients with BN, with 22.9% of monozygotic and 8.7% of dizygotic twins both diagnosed with the disorder (Kendler et al., 1991). Patients with BN are also more likely to have first-degree relatives with another eating disorder diagnosis, a substance abuse problem, an anxiety disorder, or a mood disorder, suggesting that these disorders may share common developmental pathways (Kassett et al., 1989).

Coexisting Comorbid Conditions

All of the eating disorders, including BN, commonly co-occur with other psychiatric disorders. Research indicates that nearly 82% of patients with an eating disorder have at least one concurrent Axis I disorder, while 69% meet criteria for an Axis II disorder (Braun, Sunday, & Halmi, 1994). The presence of comorbid psychopathology is of particular concern because it is associated with worse treatment outcomes (Fichter, Quadflieg, & Hedlund, 2008). Comorbid major depressive disorder is the most common lifetime Axis I diagnosis, affecting approximately 63% of individuals with BN (Brewerton et al., 1995). Although prevalence estimates vary, approximately 20% of patients with BN meet diagnostic criteria for a co-occurring substance use disorder and at least 30% meet lifetime criteria (Brewerton et al., 1995; Holderness, Brooks-Gunn, & Warren, 1994). Alcohol and substance use disorders are more often comorbid with BN than with the other eating disorders. Elevated rates of comorbid anxiety disorders also are found with BN: 68% of patients with BN have at least one anxiety disorder (Kaye, Bulik, et al., 2004). Obsessive–compulsive disorder (40%), social phobia (16%), and posttraumatic stress disorder (13%) are most common (Brewerton et al., 1995; Kaye, Bulik, et al., 2004). Posttraumatic stress disorder is significantly more common for patients with BN than AN (Kaye, Bulik, et al., 2004). Rates of the cluster B personality disorders are also elevated in patients with BN (Braun et al., 1994). Seventy percent of individuals with BN engage in some form of self-injurious behavior (Favaro & Santonastaso, 1999). BN is also associated with increased rates of childhood anxiety disorders (Kaye, Bulik, et al., 2004).

UNDERSTANDING BULIMIA NERVOSA IN COGNITIVE–BEHAVIORAL TERMS

CBT for BN is characterized by the use of a cognitive-behavioral framework for case conceptualization, as described here and expanded upon in Chapter 3, and by the use of highly structured and direct treatment interventions to disrupt the cycle of restricting, bingeing, and purging, which we describe in Chapter 4. The treatment interventions are further illustrated through a case example in Chapter 5. The explicit goals of CBT are symptom reduction and improved functioning. CBT is considered the treatment of choice for BN because there is strong empirical support for its efficacy (American Psychiatric Association, 2006). CBT may be more cost-effective than medications or other treatment modalities for the treatment of BN (Agras, 2001). Multiple

American and British medical, government, and psychological agencies recommend using CBT as the first-line treatment for BN (American Psychiatric Association, 2006; National Institute for Clinical Excellence, 2004). The following sections describe the combined behavioral, cognitive, affective, interpersonal, and emotion regulation contributors to the maintenance of BN, which are then the primary targets for treatment intervention. This conceptualization is based on the Wilson–Fairburn cognitive-behavioral model, the Cooper–Wells cognitive model, and the Fairburn transdiagnostic model of eating disorders (Cooper, Todd, & Wells, 2000; Fairburn, Cooper, & Cooper, 1986; Fairburn, Cooper, & Shafran, 2003; Wilson & Fairburn, 2002).

Behavioral Factors

Behaviors form the foundation of the cognitive-behavioral model of BN and thus are the initial focus of treatment (see Figure 2.1). The cognitive-behavioral model considers **rigid and restrictive dieting** a behavioral strategy that patients use to reduce anxiety, gain a sense of control, and achieve a preferred body shape. Strict dietary restraint, in the form of limited caloric intake, forbidden foods, and idiosyncratic dietary rules, then contributes to feelings of **deprivation and physiological hunger.** These sensations, in turn, are likely to trigger **bingeing.** Binges often consist of those foods that patients avoid at other times. The presence of "trigger" foods, combined with physical or psychological deprivation and some form of negative affect, is a common binge precipitant. Patients initially feel relief upon giving in to the urge and often experience an increase in positive affect immediately following a binge, thus reinforcing bingeing behavior (Smyth et

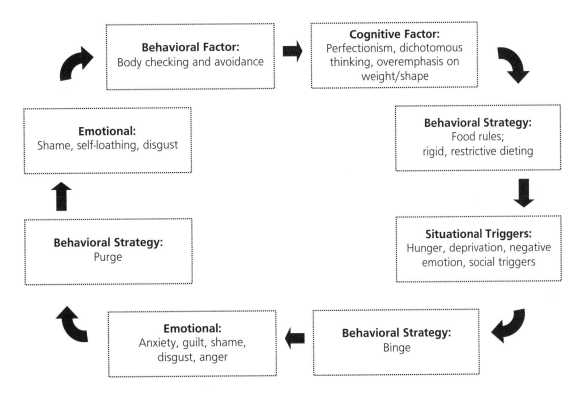

FIGURE 2.1. Cognitive-behavioral model of eating disorders.

al., 2007). As the binge continues, however, patients feel out of control, self-critical, and bloated. After a binge episode, negative affect increases, including feelings of guilt and shame (Deaver, Miltenberger, Smyth, Meidinger, & Crosby, 2003). They are then likely to **purge** in order to experience physical and emotional relief. Purging, although disliked by most patients, is reinforced as it decreases negative emotion and discomfort following the binge. Purging also gives patients a perceived "solution" to prevent weight gain from binges, thereby making future bingeing and purging more likely. Binge eating and purging form a self-maintaining cycle in which each behavior strongly predicts the other (Byrne & McLean, 2002). Following the restriction–binge–purge cycle, patients typically then vow to "try harder" and "be good" the following day, often defined as further dietary restriction. Also contributing to this behavioral cycle is **frequent weighing, body checking, and intentional body avoidance strategies,** all of which keep patients overly focused on their shape and weight (Shafran, Lee, Payne, & Fairburn, 2007).

Individuals with BN may present with highly idiosyncratic disordered eating behaviors, although there tend to be commonalities across patients. Dietary restriction, for example, may include the following: restricting caloric intake, going long periods of time without eating, eating small quantities of food throughout the day to avoid feelings of fullness, "saving up" calories for later in the day, and eliminating particular "bad" foods or entire food groups from one's diet. The dietary restriction may be reflected in patients' actual behavior, or they may have strict rules and beliefs about food to which they find it difficult to adhere. The latter is especially true in cases of BED. Because of a preoccupation with body weight and shape, patients with BN may engage in checking behaviors to monitor for any shape/weight changes. Examples of body-checking behaviors include pinching body fat, trying on "skinny" clothes, critiquing oneself in the mirror, weighing oneself multiple times daily, and frequently checking appearance in store windows. For similar reasons, individuals with BN may also actively avoid seeing their body shape or allowing it to be seen by others. They may avoid wearing fitted or revealing clothing, avoid weighing themselves, avoid looking in mirrors, avoid swimming pools and beaches, and avoid physical activities for fear of body "jiggling." These body-checking and avoidance behaviors both stem from and contribute to an overemphasis on body weight and self-critical cognitions (Shafran et al., 2007).

The first stage of CBT focuses on educating patients about and disrupting this cycle of bingeing, purging, restricting, and checking/avoidance behaviors. These behaviors are viewed as self-sabotaging but highly reinforcing choices. Behavioral change is an important aspect of treatment for BN, although research suggests that it is not effective alone (Fairburn et al., 1991).

Cognitive Factors

CBT is heavily influenced by Beck's cognitive model, which suggests that an individual's thoughts, underlying assumptions, and core beliefs determine one's behavioral and emotional reaction to a given situation (Beck, Rush, Shaw, & Emery, 1979). The broader cognitive model applies to BN, in which patients' beliefs about themselves, food, and situations maintain their problematic behaviors (Cooper et al., 2000). Patients with BN, for example, typically have low self-esteem, a high drive for thinness, and an overconcern with shape and weight (Byrne & McLean, 2002). They typically believe that their self-worth is determined wholly or largely by their body shape (Fairburn et al., 2003). These patients, therefore, spend a great deal of time thinking, often negatively, about their body weight and food intake (Alvarenga, Scagliusi, & Philippi, 2008; Cash & Deagle, 1997). Patients with BN also hold more negative core beliefs related to their self-worth, success, self-control, lovability, and physical attractiveness than other people (Somerville & Cooper, 2007). For example, patients often believe that they are only attractive and lovable if they are thin enough, and may equate dieting with "goodness" and "control." These cognitions influence patients' continued restrictive dieting and body-checking behaviors. Patients also hold rigid rules about food ("Potato chips are bad and, therefore, completely off limits"), their diets ("I should never eat between meals"), and weight gain ("I gained 5 pounds after overeating at one meal") (Alvarenga et al., 2008). When one of these food rules is broken, patients are likely to interpret this as having "blown it," to "give up," and to then binge (Cooper et al., 2000). Patients typically equate bingeing with "failure" and personal weakness, triggering further self-criticism and a desire to reverse the perceived consequences of the binge. Purging and the remainder of the cycle then follow, including continued overemphasis on weight and shape.

Just as with the behavioral factors, patients with BN often share similar negative thought patterns that help maintain their eating disorder (see Table 2.1). Patients may hold the **core beliefs** of "I am worthless," "I am flawed," and "I am unlovable." A compensatory rule, or **underlying assumption,** stemming from these core beliefs may be, "I am only worthwhile and lovable

TABLE 2.1. Sample Cognitions in Bulimia Nervosa

Automatic thoughts	Underlying assumptions	Core schemas
"They won't hire me because I'm too fat."	"I am only attractive if I am thin."	"I am unattractive."
"I should skip lunch to compensate for last night's binge."	"If I don't restrict my eating, everything will spiral out of control."	"I am out of control."
"Karen thinks I am an emotional wreck."	"If I express my emotions to others, they will see me as a burden."	"I am a burden."
"I will probably get fired after screwing up that report for my boss."	"If I make mistakes, no one will respect me."	"I am incompetent."
"I should not eat in front of people at this party. They will think I am a pig."	"If I don't keep everything in control, people will see that I'm a failure."	"I am a failure."
"Bob is going to leave me."	"If I ever disagree or there is a conflict, the relationship will end."	"I am vulnerable." "Others are unreliable."
"My husband must think I am so weak and crazy."	"If I don't present myself perfectly, people will see me as weird."	"I am weird." "I am flawed."

if I am thin." Seen through the lens of these underlying beliefs, patients with BN may then mis-interpret a situation with a negative **automatic thought** ("I was passed over for my job promotion because I'm too fat. I can't get anything right"). Patients' thoughts are typically characterized by self-criticism, negativity, rigidity, fear of losing control, and perfectionism. Cognitive therapists have also observed that patients hold positive beliefs about their bingeing, purging, and dietary restriction, all of which equally contribute to the eating disorder cycle (Cooper, Wells, & Todd, 2004). Positive thoughts may include "Cutting out certain foods entirely helps me to stay in control"; "I will feel better if I purge to get rid of this binge"; "Binges are soothing"; "I've had a stressful day, so I deserve to eat potato chips"; and "Urges never go away, so I have to give in and binge."

Cognitive factors maintain patients' poor body image, dietary rigidity, perceived inability to resist urges to binge, and other eating disorder behaviors. If left unchallenged or untested, these cognitions also make patients more vulnerable to posttreatment relapse. Thus, the second stage of treatment is to address these cognitions. This cognitive phase of treatment starts with the identification and testing of patients' problematic automatic thoughts, underlying assump-tions, and core beliefs. Ultimately, the goal is to replace these thought patterns with more func-tional and balanced beliefs. Adoption of less biased and more flexible cognitions further helps to decrease bingeing and purging, improves self-esteem, and allows for more flexible food- and weight-related self-standards. It is worth noting that cognitive-behavioral treatment focuses on changing the behaviors and beliefs occurring in the present, and early childhood experiences are a focus of treatment only in helping to clarify how they have contributed to patients' current assumptions and beliefs.

Interpersonal Factors

Fairburn and colleagues (2003) described interpersonal factors as additional maintaining mecha-nisms for BN. Supporting the stated importance of interpersonal factors, IPT is considered to be as effective as CBT for BN, although the positive outcomes may take longer to achieve (National Institute for Clinical Excellence, 2004). Additionally, some practitioners have effectively com-bined CBT and IPT in the treatment of eating disorders (Fairburn et al., 2009; Hendricks & Thompson, 2005). Problematic interpersonal factors can directly or indirectly influence eating disorder behaviors through the promotion of rigid ideals for thinness; modeling of bingeing and dieting behaviors; interpersonal comparisons, social isolation, fears of rejection; and situational stressors that precipitate negative affect, bingeing, and dieting (Wilfley et al., 1993). These factors may include, but are not limited to, the following: standards for thinness and appearance within one's social network, family, or profession; a culture of restrictive dieting among one's friends; friends or family members with eating disorders; a social norm for using shape and appearance to obtain approval; social isolation and lack of social support; social skills deficits; problematic thoughts and feelings in interpersonal situations; difficulties with assertiveness; interpersonal conflict or tensions; and role transitions (e.g., leaving for college or getting married). Throughout CBT, a patient's unique interpersonal difficulties will be identified and addressed as they affect BN behaviors, cognitive beliefs, and lack of effective coping skills. The same main interpersonal problem areas that are addressed in IPT for BN are incorporated into this cognitive-behavioral treatment: grief; interpersonal disputes; problematic thoughts, feelings, and emotions in interpersonal relationships; role transitions; lack of assertiveness; and interpersonal deficits (Arcelus et al., 2009; Wilfley et al., 1993).

A common interpersonal trigger for patients with BN involves food and hunger norms that are set by their friends, which contribute to binge eating and dietary restriction. For example, a patient often socializes with her friends in the evening after work. Her friends overtly avoid consuming full meals. Several appetizers are ordered and, while the patient remains hungry, her friends comment that they are "so full." The patient feels guilty and ashamed for seemingly requiring more food than others, and she labels herself negatively as a result. After the patient leaves her friends and arrives home, she is left vulnerable to bingeing because she is hungry, emotional, consumed with negative thinking, and alone. The more this patient binges after dining with her friends, the more out of control and ashamed she feels. She may then avoid going out with her friends in the evening to prevent bingeing, or she may engage in an ongoing pattern of secretive eating, interpersonal anxiety, and periods of dietary restriction. This resulting pattern of behavior then exacerbates the patient's interpersonal problems, including grief, social isolation, and interpersonal conflict.

Emotion Regulation

Throughout the cognitive-behavioral cycle of BN, the role of emotion and poor distress tolerance is apparent. Strong emotional states, whether positive or negative, may precede and follow the eating disorder behavior. Specifically, binge eating often follows a rise in negative affect, anger, and stress, and bingeing has been shown to temporarily alleviate this negative affective state (Smyth et al., 2007). Shortly after the binge, however, the negative emotional state is worse than before the binge (Wegner et al., 2002). It is likely that the original negative emotion not only returns shortly after the binge, but is exacerbated by feelings of fullness, shame, and self-loathing from the binge.

An inability to tolerate, moderate, or effectively express affective states may make the patient with BN particularly vulnerable to bingeing, purging, and distorted cognitions, which are thought to be maladaptive behavioral attempts at affect regulation (Deaver et al., 2003). In turn, bingeing, purging, negative automatic thoughts, and interpersonal situations may spur negative emotion, such as depression or anxiety, further contributing to the cyclical nature of BN. Preliminary research suggests that teaching emotion regulation and self-soothing skills to patients with BN significantly reduces episodes of bingeing and purging (Esplen, Garfinkel, Olmsted, Gallop, & Kennedy, 1998; Safer et al., 2001). Emotional dysregulation and mood intolerance are thought to be contributors to eating disorder behaviors, and thus it is recommended that CBT help patients identify their emotional states, safely express their emotion, develop effective coping skills to tolerate strong emotions, and learn alternative strategies to ameliorate negative mood states (Deaver et al., 2003; Fairburn et al., 2003).

Treatment Outcome Research

CBT for BN has been shown to be more effective than supportive psychotherapies, psychoeducational groups, and dynamic-oriented therapy (Lewandowski, Gebing, Anthony, & O'Brien, 1997; Shapiro et al., 2007; Walsh et al., 1997; Whittal, Agras, & Gould, 1999). CBT also is more effective than medications alone and may produce a more rapid reduction in dieting and purging than IPT (Agras, Walsh, et al., 2000; Mitchell et al., 1990). CBT effectively eliminates binge eating and purging in 40–50% of individuals who complete treatment, and patients' abstinence has been shown to be stable over time (Wilson, Fairburn, & Agras, 1997). Even among those who do not achieve complete remission with CBT, many experience improvement in their BN symptoms. At least 75% show a reduction in bingeing and purging and an evident improvement in body image (Wilson et al., 1997).

There is no single factor that contributes to treatment success, but there are multiple factors that have been shown to be positive or negative predictors of treatment outcome. Individuals who make significant gains within the first 4 weeks of CBT, specifically in elimination or reduction of purging behaviors, are most likely to fully recover (Agras, Crow, et al., 2000; Fairburn, Agras, Walsh, Wilson, & Stice, 2004). In addition, patients who view CBT as a logical treatment are more likely to remain engaged, and those with a positive view of the therapeutic alliance are more likely to recover (Wilson et al., 1999). Together, these findings suggest the importance of a full explanation of the CBT model and treatment rationale to the patients, the development of excellent rapport early in treatment, and a focus on behavior change in the early treatment sessions. Negative predictors of treatment outcome include longer duration of illness, greater comorbid depressive symptoms, comorbid Axis II psychopathology, a history of substance abuse or dependence, more impulsivity, low body weight, more frequent purging, and severe dietary restriction at the start of treatment (Agras, Crow, et al., 2000; Fairburn et al., 2004; Reas, Williamson, Martin, & Zucker, 2000; Wilson et al., 1999). Despite the potential for greater difficulty during treatment, individuals with any of the listed negative predictors may still benefit and fully recover with CBT for BN.

PSYCHOTROPIC MEDICATIONS FOR EATING DISORDERS

The therapist treating patients with eating disorders will often work in collaboration with a full treatment team, including an internist, psychopharmacologist, and nutritionist, and therefore a basic understanding of the types, doses, and efficacy of psychotropic medications is helpful. Fluoxetine, a selective serotonin reuptake inhibitor (SSRI), is the only medication approved by the U.S. Food and Drug Administration for the treatment of BN, and its suggested therapeutic dose (60 mg/day) is higher than that used for major depression (American Psychiatric Association, 2006). Sertraline, another SSRI antidepressant, and desipramine, a tricyclic antidepressant, have also been shown to be effective. Antidepressant medication alone rarely leads to full remission of BN symptoms, and the use of antidepressants is associated with higher dropout rates from psychological treatments as a result of medication side effects (American Psychiatric Association, 2006; Mitchell et al., 2007). With medication treatment alone, patients with BN or BED tend to relapse to binge eating once the medication is discontinued. If patients are to respond well to treatment with antidepressant medication, significant improvement in BN symptoms is typically apparent within 2–4 weeks (Walsh, Sysko, & Parides, 2005). The most commonly reported side effects for fluoxetine are sexual side effects, insomnia, and nausea. Because of the risk of seizures associated with purging behavior, buproprion is contraindicated for patients with BN or purging disorder.

Limited treatment research has been conducted to date on psychotropic medications for BED. Several SSRIs, tricyclic antipressants, and topiramate, an anticonvulsant, have shown promising results in reducing the frequency of binges (American Psychiatric Association, 2006; Reas & Grilo, 2008). As in BN, the recommended therapeutic dosage for medications for BED is at the high end of the recommended range (American Psychiatric Association, 2006). The SSRIs and tricyclic antidepressants do not help patients with BED achieve significant weight loss. However, topiramate and sibutramine, a serotonin–norepinephrine reuptake inhibitor, may positively affect both binge eating and body weight (McElroy et al., 2003; Wilfley et al., 2008).

Despite the greater risk of premature termination of treatment, providing concurrent antidepressant medication and CBT for eating disorders may be most effective (Agras, 1997). This is especially true for patients presenting with depressive symptoms, those exhibiting poor initial response to cognitive-behavioral interventions, and those with greater impulsivity (American Psychiatric Association, 2006). Some research suggests that patients with BN show more improvement in binge eating and depressive symptoms when CBT is combined with an antidepressant (Agras et al., 1992; Walsh et al., 1997).

CHAPTER 3

Assessment, Diagnosis, and Treatment Planning

A careful assessment of the patient is necessary at the outset of treatment to determine the appropriate level of care, to educate the patient about her eating disorder, and to formulate an individualized treatment plan. Assessment typically occurs during the first three treatment sessions, and ideally is done collaboratively with the patient in order to develop good rapport and to set the tone for the remainder of treatment. CBT is not conducted by simply matching therapeutic interventions to patient symptoms, but instead is defined by using a cognitive-behavioral case conceptualization to guide treatment. The case conceptualization and subsequent treatment plan are developed following a thorough assessment of the patient's presenting problems, symptom history, comorbid psychopathology, and maladaptive cognitions (automatic thoughts, assumptions/conditional rules, personal schemas). As described in Chapter 2, the integrative approach advanced in this book also includes emotional regulation, interpersonal issues, and developmental history (where relevant) in the case conceptualization. Case conceptualization can also include consideration of personal strengths, coping skills deficits, and resources available. During formal assessment, the therapist should consult the diagnostic flow chart for BN (Figure 3.1) and the Evaluation of Eating Disorders (see Form B.1, Evaluation of Eating Disorders, in Appendix B). The Eating Disorders Examination Questionnaire (EDE-Q, see Form B.2), the Clinical Impairment Assessment Questionnaire (see Form B.3), the Body Image Checklist (see Form B.4), the Eating Disorder Belief Questionnaire (see Form B.5), BMI charts for adults (see Form B.6) and adolescents (see Form B.7), and the Evaluation of Suicide Risk (see Form B.8) are included in Appendix B. These assessment instruments can be useful to assess the presence and severity of symptoms at intake and to monitor the patient's improvement over the course of treatment.

Following formal assessment, the therapist should provide the patient with feedback about the severity of her symptoms relative to others with and without an eating disorder, review the current and potential consequences of her eating disorder, and outline the expected course of treatment. It is often useful to reference the patient's scores on the self-report assessments and to explain whether these scores are within or above the normal range (see Appendix B). For example, the therapist may explain to the patient that her twice-daily use of laxatives is particularly dangerous and suggests a more extreme eating disorder, and that this behavior will be targeted

Is the patient . . . ?

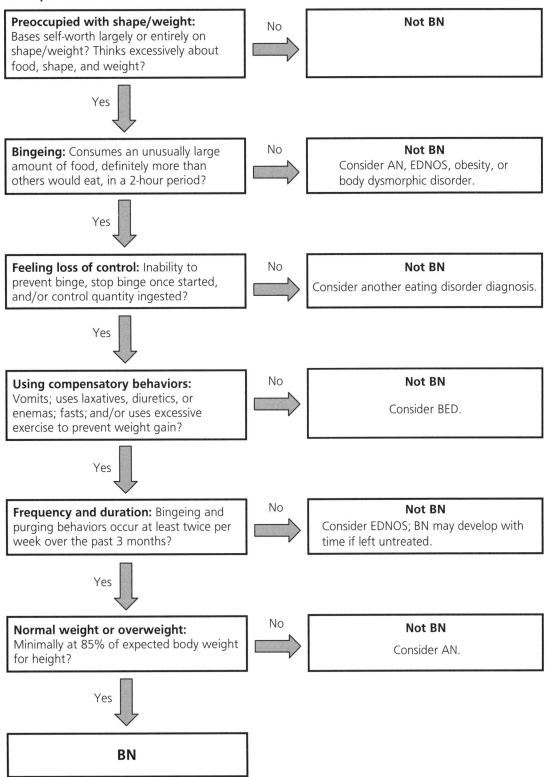

FIGURE 3.1. Diagnostic flow chart for bulimia nervosa.

immediately in treatment. Additionally, the therapist may review the patient's assessment scores, giving feedback that her mood is in the moderately depressed range (Beck Depression Inventory [BDI] score = 23, where 20–28 is considered moderately depressed) and her weight is below normal, suggesting she is engaging in significant dietary restriction (BMI = 19, where 20–24 is considered healthy). Patient education and orientation to cognitive-behavioral treatment also can be facilitated by discussing the cognitive-behavioral model of eating disorders, showing how the behaviors, cognitions, and triggers endorsed during the assessment phase fit in to this model (see Figure 2.1). The therapist can also provide the patient with a handout that briefly outlines what to expect during treatment (Form 3.1).

DIFFERENTIAL DIAGNOSIS

Only one eating disorder can be diagnosed at a time, and AN always takes diagnostic precedence. **AN** is characterized by an intense fear of and a refusal to maintain a normal body weight. Severe dietary restriction and/or purging may be intentionally used to maintain a low body weight. Disruption in one's menstrual cycle is also a distinguishing feature of AN. **BN** is marked by frequent binge eating followed by purging or other unhealthy compensatory behaviors. Patients with BN are preoccupied with their body shape, often engage in extreme dieting between binges to obtain a low body weight, and feel a loss of control and intense distress related to their bingeing. When eating disorder symptoms are sufficiently extreme to cause impairment and distress but do not meet diagnostic criteria for either AN or BN, **EDNOS** is diagnosed. Although it is designed to be a residual category for eating disorders, EDNOS is the most common of the eating disorders diagnoses, accounting for 40–60% of all cases (Button, Benson, Nollett, & Palmer, 2005; Fairburn et al., 2007). EDNOS is also the least studied of all eating disorder diagnoses. Most cases of EDNOS are individuals with mixed eating disorder symptoms, although subthreshold AN or BN would also fall under EDNOS. Thus, EDNOS could include an individual with all but one of the symptoms required for AN or BN; an individual who has all symptoms of AN or BN but does not meet minimum frequency or duration criteria; purging disorder; and BED. **Purging disorder** is a variant of BN in which individuals do not binge but consistently purge following ingestion of "subjective binges" or normal quantities of food. **BED** is characterized by repeated episodes of binge eating (without purging) that result in significant distress for the patient. Although they are both currently diagnosed under EDNOS, recent research suggests that purging disorder and BED are both significant psychological disorders distinct from BN (Keel, 2007; Latner & Clyne, 2008). All of the eating disorders, including EDNOS, are serious mental illnesses and may result in significant psychological and/or medical consequences.

Body weight alone is not a definitive diagnostic tool, although it may differ among patients with eating disorders. Patients with AN are, by definition, significantly underweight, and they must also display other significant symptoms of this disorder. Patients with BN are often at a normal body weight, although they may be slightly underweight or overweight. The body weight of patients with BED varies considerably; however, many patients are significantly overweight and often present for weight loss treatment.

Individuals who meet diagnostic criteria for AN cannot also receive a BN or EDNOS diagnosis. Those who have lost weight rapidly, who exhibit abnormal eating behavior, or who frequently vomit as a result of a medical condition or substance use, but who do not exhibit preoccupation with shape and weight, would not receive an eating disorder diagnosis. Individuals who regularly purge or use other compensatory behaviors in the absence of binges, such as after eating regular meals or consuming small quantities of food, do not meet the criteria for BN. A diagnosis of AN (purging type) should be considered. Refer to the diagnostic flow chart for BN (Figure 3.1).

It has been suggested that a large number of patients presenting for eating disorders treatment in the community will not meet the diagnostic criteria for BN but that approximately 50–75% will instead meet criteria for EDNOS (Machado, Machado, Gonçalves, & Hock, 2007; Ricca et al., 2001). EDNOS encompasses eating disorders that occur on the continuum between AN and BN, eating disorders with purging but without bingeing behaviors, BED, "subjective" binges only (no objectively large consumption of food), and bingeing and purging that does not meet diagnostic criteria for frequency or duration. EDNOS may closely resemble BN and can be characterized by the same psychopathological and maintaining factors as BN: rigidity, perfectionism, extreme attention to weight and shape, and bingeing and purging (Fairburn et al., 2003; Ricca et al., 2001). These shared symptoms and clinical presentations across the eating disorders further support the utility of Fairburn's transdiagnostic model of the eating disorders (see Appendix A). In addition, the traditional CBT for BN, which is presented in this book, may be appropriate for those patients with EDNOS who share clinical features and symptoms with BN.

TREATMENT PLANNING

At this stage, the therapist should ascertain what level of treatment is appropriate for the patient. Level-of-care decisions, as discussed in Chapter 1, are based on prior treatment history and outcomes, severity of current BN symptoms, medical status, and comorbid psychiatric conditions. The included decision tree can help the therapist ascertain the appropriate level of care for patients with eating disorders (see Figure 3.2).

Suicide is a considerable risk, with suicide attempts occurring in 11–40% of patients with BN. The therapist should carefully assess for suicidality at the outset of treatment and throughout the course of treatment, because psychotherapy may not alleviate the risk of suicide (Franko et al., 2004). Risk factors for suicide among patients with BN, which include a history of or concurrent alcohol or substance abuse, laxative use, impulsivity, comorbid borderline personality disorder, paranoia and greater mistrust of others, prior sexual abuse, significant depression, and an earlier age of onset of BN, should have been assessed at the outset of treatment and will influence the level of treatment suggested by the therapist (Bulik, Sullivan, Carter, & Joyce, 1997; Corcos et al., 2002; Franko et al., 2004; see Appendix B.8 and Form B.8). In short, those patients presenting with the most severe and complex psychopathology may be at greatest risk for suicide.

Medical and dental complications of BN are a considerable risk for patients and are most often associated with low body weight or purging, including the use of vomiting, laxatives, or diuretics (Agras, 2001; American Psychiatric Association, 2006; Anderson, 1992; Mehler & Anderson, 2000). Potential medical and dental risks associated with BN are described in Table 3.1. The most common consequences of BN are dental erosion, swelling of the salivary glands, dry skin, low blood pressure, and slowed heart rate (Mehler, Birmingham, Crow, & Jahraus, 2010). Patients with BN may also exhibit "Russell's sign," or the characteristic callusing of the back of

Does the patient . . . ?

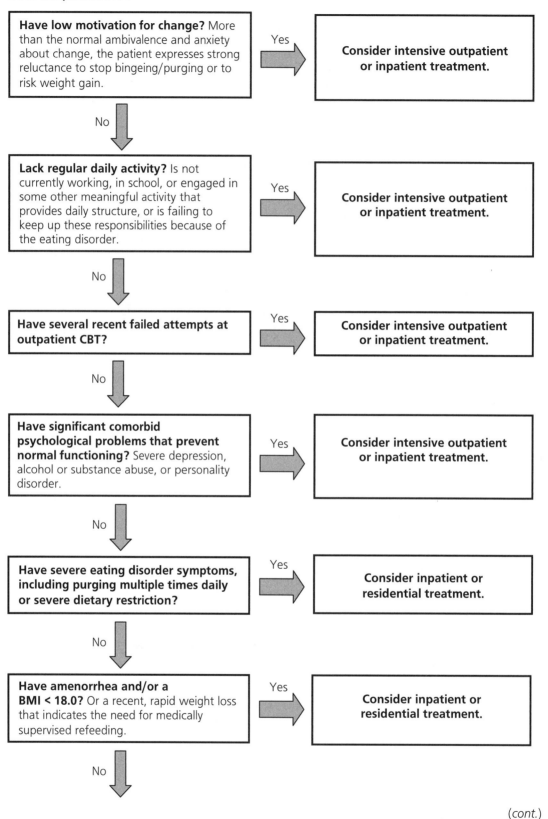

Have low motivation for change? More than the normal ambivalence and anxiety about change, the patient expresses strong reluctance to stop bingeing/purging or to risk weight gain.

Yes → **Consider intensive outpatient or inpatient treatment.**

No ↓

Lack regular daily activity? Is not currently working, in school, or engaged in some other meaningful activity that provides daily structure, or is failing to keep up these responsibilities because of the eating disorder.

Yes → **Consider intensive outpatient or inpatient treatment.**

No ↓

Have several recent failed attempts at outpatient CBT?

Yes → **Consider intensive outpatient or inpatient treatment.**

No ↓

Have significant comorbid psychological problems that prevent normal functioning? Severe depression, alcohol or substance abuse, or personality disorder.

Yes → **Consider intensive outpatient or inpatient treatment.**

No ↓

Have severe eating disorder symptoms, including purging multiple times daily or severe dietary restriction?

Yes → **Consider inpatient or residential treatment.**

No ↓

Have amenorrhea and/or a BMI < 18.0? Or a recent, rapid weight loss that indicates the need for medically supervised refeeding.

Yes → **Consider inpatient or residential treatment.**

No ↓

(cont.)

FIGURE 3.2. Level-of-care decision tree for eating disorders.

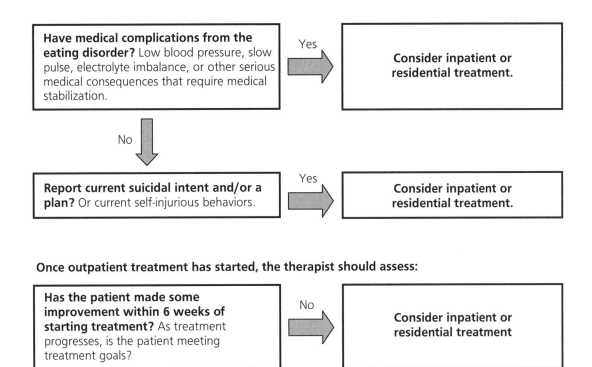

<table>
<tr><td>

Have medical complications from the eating disorder? Low blood pressure, slow pulse, electrolyte imbalance, or other serious medical consequences that require medical stabilization.

</td><td>Yes →</td><td>

Consider inpatient or residential treatment.

</td></tr>
</table>

No ↓

<table>
<tr><td>

Report current suicidal intent and/or a plan? Or current self-injurious behaviors.

</td><td>Yes →</td><td>

Consider inpatient or residential treatment.

</td></tr>
</table>

Once outpatient treatment has started, the therapist should assess:

<table>
<tr><td>

Has the patient made some improvement within 6 weeks of starting treatment? As treatment progresses, is the patient meeting treatment goals?

</td><td>No →</td><td>

Consider inpatient or residential treatment

</td></tr>
</table>

FIGURE 3.2 (*cont.*)

the hands caused by self-induced vomiting (Mehler et al., 2010). Fortunately, fatal complications are uncommon among patients with BN. Life-threatening medical complications include cardiac arrest and esophageal rupture. When fatalities occur, they are usually due to cardiac problems (associated with purging) or suicide. Electrolyte imbalance can result from loss of fluids associated with vomiting, laxative use, or diuretic use. The most common electrolyte imbalance in patients with BN is hypokalemia, or low serum potassium levels, although chloride, sodium, and bicarbonate levels can also be affected.

At treatment intake, the therapist should refer the patient to an internist to ascertain medical stability, to rule out electrolyte imbalance and other serious medical complications, and to monitor vital signs. The physician typically performs laboratory blood tests and checks the patient's body weight, blood pressure, pulse, hydration levels, and constipation at this examination. Laboratory tests can identify hyperamylasemia (elevated blood amylase levels, thought to be associated with frequent vomiting), hypokalemia (low blood levels of potassium), and metabolic alkalosis (pH imbalance typically resulting from vomiting) in the patient. These conditions, although serious, are rare and may not be present in even the most severe cases of an eating disorder. If the eating disorder is severe or longstanding or cardiac damage is suspected, the physician may order an electrocardiogram. Continuous medical monitoring is warranted throughout treatment, preferably on a weekly basis and especially in the presence of continued purging, severe dietary restriction, any abnormal vital signs or blood tests, or underweight. In these cases, the therapist will need to advise the patient to have weekly blood tests completed by the physician, and the patient should bring the therapist a copy of the laboratory results. Once the patient signs a written release of information, the therapist can communicate directly with the physician

TABLE 3.1. Medical and Dental Risks Associated with Bulimia Nervosa

Possible medical consequences from restricted food intake, vomiting, laxative use, and/or low body weight:

- Abdominal bloating or cramping
- Acid reflux
- Anemia
- Arrhythmia (irregular heartbeat)
- Chronic constipation
- Dehydration
- Dizziness
- Electrolyte imbalance (elevated or decreased serum potassium, sodium, bicarbonate, or chloride levels)
- Esophageal inflammation and damage
- Fatigue
- Gastrointestinal bleeding
- Heart failure
- Hyperamylasemia (elevated levels of amylase, a digestive enzyme)
- Irritable bowel syndrome
- Kidney failure
- Low blood pressure
- Menstrual irregularities or amenorrhea
- Metabolic alkalosis (elevated blood pH levels)
- Pancreatitis
- Seizures
- Slowed pulse rate
- Sore throat
- Swelling of hands and feet
- Swollen parotid (salivary) glands (resulting in swollen cheeks)
- Ulcers

Common dental consequences from vomiting:

- Cavities
- Cheilosis (scaling and sores at corners of the mouth)
- Erosion of dental enamel
- Gingivitis
- Mouth ulcers
- Periodontal disease
- Sensitivity to hot and cold foods
- Tooth loss

---

to discuss the expected frequency of vital signs and laboratory testing, to receive results, and to update one another on improvement or setbacks in the patient's symptoms. Typically, the patient is compliant with medical monitoring, especially when the therapist outlines the potential medical complications of BN that require monitoring and prevention. If the patient resists medical monitoring, the therapist should treat this like any other noncompliance in treatment (see Chapter 4, Possible "Roadblocks" and Treatment Resistance section). Clearly, ongoing professional consultation between the therapist and the internist, often in the form of brief weekly telephone calls or e-mails, is important to guarantee the patient's safety and optimal care.

Case Conceptualization

After a thorough intake assessment, the cognitive-behavioral therapist should develop a detailed case conceptualization for the patient (see Form 3.2). The Case Conceptualization Worksheet is completed by and intended primarily for use by the therapist, although the therapist can use clinical judgment to decide when to share the worksheet with the patient. Case conceptualization is a tool to ensure that the therapist views the patient's eating disorder and comorbid psychological problems in a manner consistent with the cognitive-behavioral model (described in Chapter 2). The case conceptualization also helps the therapist attend to all behavioral, cognitive, interpersonal, situational, and emotional symptoms when setting treatment goals, planning the course of treatment, and evaluating treatment progress. Thus, the therapist will generate the case conceptualization prior to the start of active treatment sessions, but should also regularly review the case conceptualization throughout treatment.

Typically, the cognitive-behavioral therapist completes the case conceptualization worksheet for each patient between the assessment and initial treatment sessions, although it may require updating as new clinical information arises over the course of treatment. This case conceptualization will include cognitions, behaviors, and symptoms specific to the patient's eating disorder and any comorbid psychological problems. The therapist will gather this information through the Evaluation of Eating Disorders, other intake assessment measures, and the patient's description of her presenting problems. The presence and frequency of bingeing and purging, queried on both the Evaluation of Eating Disorders and the EDE-Q, will be recorded in their respective places on the case conceptualization. The Evaluation of Eating Disorders also generates the patient's self-described food rules, negative cognitions, thoughts related to body image, and emotional and situational triggers for eating disorder symptoms, all of which will be included in the case conceptualization in the appropriate place. Any elevated subscale scores on the intake assessment measures indicate problems that need to be addressed in treatment, and these scores should also be recorded on the case conceptualization. For example, a patient with elevated Eating Concern or Weight Concern subscale scores on the EDE-Q shows cognitive factors maintaining the eating disorder. It is worth reiterating the importance of including all behavioral, cognitive, and emotional symptoms in the case conceptualization, not simply those factors the patient identifies as distressing (e.g, views bingeing as problematic but wants to retain a rigid diet). A sample completed case conceptualization is provided with the case example in Chapter 5.

The case conceptualization is then used to guide the therapist's treatment planning, linking present symptoms, thoughts, and emotions to specific cognitive-behavioral interventions. The case conceptualization also helps the therapist to attend first to the most acute and dangerous psychopathology as well as to recognize the presence of comorbid disorders that will prevent progress in eating disorder treatment (i.e., stabilize suicidal depression before beginning treatment of moderately severe BN; treat current alcohol abuse before or concurrently with severe BN; treat BN before generalized anxiety disorder). In some instances when thought to be clinically useful, the case conceptualization may be shared with the patient as part of the orientation to treatment. However, the case conceptualization is primarily intended to be a tool for the therapist to help ensure adherence to the cognitive-behavioral model while addressing the patient's unique presenting symptoms and thought patterns.

Individualized Treatment Planning

Although the treatment plan for BN, described in Chapter 4, is appropriate for all patients with BN, the therapist may need to tailor the treatment goals, interventions used, and pace of treatment to match each patient's presenting symptoms, unique situational triggers, degree of motivation, idiosyncratic food rules, and any psychiatric, medical, or interpersonal comorbidity. A thorough intake assessment, a functional analysis of binge–purge triggers, and a detailed case conceptualization will guide the therapist in individualizing treatment for each patient. A solid understanding of the patient's eating disorder, combined with good clinical judgment, will allow the therapist to tailor this treatment plan for each individual.

Thorough intake assessment, collaborative goal setting, orientation to the cognitive-behavioral model, psychoeducation about eating disorders, daily food records, motivational enhancement, regular eating, cognitive restructuring, and relapse prevention will be used with all patients with eating disorders. The interpersonal and emotional interventions, however, are designed to be optional components of treatment. Other cognitive-behavioral interventions described in the treatment plan may be omitted, expanded upon, or adapted depending on the therapist's case conceptualization for the patient. For example, some patients with BN will engage in particularly long periods of dietary restriction with only sporadic eating and, therefore, treatment will need to emphasize regular eating. For these patients, regular eating may be the focus of multiple treatment sessions rather than the one to two sessions described in the treatment plan. A particular focus on selected treatment interventions will be in addition to, not in lieu of, the other cognitive-behavioral interventions in the treatment plan. Other patients with BN may exhibit a very strong fear of weight gain and a desire to maintain a dangerously low body weight. In that case, the therapist will need to spend considerable time educating them about the cognitive-behavioral model of eating disorders, give repeated feedback about current and expected body weight, set weight gain as a treatment goal, challenge unrealistic standards and negative cognitions about body weight, redefine healthy, and spend additional time on the body image interventions included in this treatment plan. For some patients with a particularly low body weight, weight gain may need to be a condition for outpatient treatment, and a failure to gain weight may warrant referral to a higher level of treatment. Other patients will receive the cognitive-behavioral treatment just as described in Chapter 4 until experiencing a setback or full relapse to eating disorder symptoms. At that time, the therapist and patients will need to return to relevant prior interventions and extend the overall length of treatment.

Adapting Treatment for Eating Disorder Not Otherwise Specified

The treatment plan described in Chapter 4 can also be readily adapted for use with patients with BED, purging disorder, or another variant of EDNOS. Although each eating disorder has distinct symptoms, there is considerable overlap of their cognitive, behavioral, and emotional symptoms. Most patients with an eating disorder, regardless of diagnosis, experience similar cognitive factors (e.g., perfectionism and dichotomous thinking), a preoccupation with body weight and shape, an intense fear of weight gain, rigid food rules, and fear of certain foods or food groups. In addition, most attempt to restrict their diets, have insufficient emotional coping skills, and engage in some form of body checking or avoidance. The cognitive-behavioral treatment plan included in this book addresses each of these common factors for the eating disorders.

The treatment goals for all patients with eating disorders, regardless of diagnosis, include normalizing eating patterns, reducing preoccupation with shape/weight, and improving daily functioning. Additional treatment goals will be dependent on the patient's presenting symptoms and the therapist's case conceptualization for her. On the basis of the case conceptualization and the collaborative treatment goals, the therapist will select the specific interventions to be used throughout treatment. For example, a patient with purging disorder may vomit after eating normal meals or after consuming any quantity of a "forbidden food." Because this patient does not binge, the therapist will not need to incorporate stimulus control measures aimed at reducing binge triggers. However, psychoeducation about the dangers of purging, developing alternative activities to purging, and practicing "urge surfing" will be a primary focus of treatment. In addition, the therapist will need to help this patient challenge dichotomized and catastrophic thinking about food intake and to normalize the patient's diet through regular eating and reincorporating restricted foods. Thus, the treatment will progress largely according to the treatment plan described in Chapter 4, although cognitive and behavioral interventions will target dietary restriction and purging, not bingeing.

Another patient with a diagnosis of EDNOS and whose symptoms are consistent with BED can also receive an adapted form of the treatment plan. This patient's case conceptualization will reflect a strong preoccupation with body weight, repeated attempts at dieting, numerous "bad" foods, self-loathing related to being overweight, multiple forms of body checking and avoidance, and bingeing most nights because of loneliness and fatigue. However, this patient does not purge. The only evident compensatory behavior is a tendency to skip breakfast the morning after a binge. The treatment plan for a patient with BED will be nearly identical to that of a patient with BN, although no interventions for purging will be necessary. All other psychoeducational, cognitive, behavioral, body image, and relapse prevention interventions will help this patient normalize daily eating patterns, decrease preoccupation with body weight, discontinue bingeing, challenge unrealistic and destructive thoughts related to food and body image, and develop more adaptive emotional coping skills.

To meet the diagnostic criteria for BN, a patient must binge and purge at least twice weekly for a 3-month period. A patient who exhibits all other cognitive and behavioral symptoms of BN, including a clear negative impact on daily functioning, but who binges and purges once weekly would receive a diagnosis of EDNOS. This patient still has a serious eating disorder that requires treatment. A therapist's case conceptualization for this patient would look nearly identical to that of a patient with BN, and the entire treatment described in Chapter 4 would be applicable. The treatment would be personalized for the patient's unique cognitions, food rules, binge triggers, and comorbidities, as described previously, but no other adjustments would need to be made for subthreshold BN.

As is clear from the prior examples, patients with any eating disorder diagnosis, as long as they are not critically underweight, can benefit from a customized form of the outpatient cognitive-behavioral treatment described in Chapter 4.

FORM 3.1. Information for Patients about Bulimia Nervosa

WHAT IS BULIMIA NERVOSA?

The symptoms most associated with bulimia nervosa are bingeing, purging, and a preoccupation with shape and body weight. If you consume an objectively large amount of food in a relatively short amount of time, this is called a *binge*. During a binge, a person typically eats very rapidly, feels *out of control*, and feels unable to stop eating. You may feel emotionally numb, shut down, or "outside yourself" while bingeing. Binges typically occur in secret, and they are usually followed by feelings of disgust, physical discomfort, and shame. To compensate for the binge and a fear of gaining weight, individuals with bulimia nervosa will *purge*, *exercise excessively*, or *fast* (e.g., skip breakfast and lunch the day following an evening binge). Purging is the term used to describe intentional vomiting, laxative use, diuretic use, and use of enemas after bingeing. As an eating disorder becomes more severe, individuals may purge even after normal meals or after ingesting small amounts of food. *Preoccupation with shape and weight* is another defining symptom of bulimia nervosa. You may find that you spend most of your time thinking about food and weight, are intensely afraid of gaining weight, repeatedly pinch your "problem areas," check yourself in mirrors, weigh yourself obsessively, try on "skinny" clothes to check your weight, feel upset or anxious when you are full, and base your self-worth almost entirely on your shape and weight.

If you are struggling with bulimia nervosa, you probably also experience some or all of the following symptoms: have strict, inflexible *dietary rules*; have many forbidden foods; label foods as "good" or "bad"; eat in secret; hide food; avoid eating or socializing with friends; and feel disgusted by your body.

People struggling with bulimia nervosa may be normal weight, slightly underweight, or overweight. Bulimia nervosa affects men and women, individuals of all races and socioeconomic backgrounds, athletes and nonathletes, and adolescents and adults.

WHAT CAUSES BULIMIA NERVOSA?

Bulimia nervosa affects approximately 2% of the population. The exact cause of bulimia nervosa is unknown, although it likely results from a complex combination of multiple factors. Biology, psychological vulnerabilities, learned thinking patterns and behaviors, familial experiences, and societal pressures all likely play a part in the development of bulimia nervosa. If a parent or sibling has had problems with eating disorders, obesity, alcoholism, substance abuse, depression, or anxiety, you may have had elevated risk of developing an eating disorder.

What we do know is that the causes of an eating disorder may be different from the factors maintaining the problem. In short, once developed, the eating disorder takes on a life of its own. The behaviors and thinking patterns that are addressed in cognitive-behavioral therapy are those same factors that maintain the eating disorder.

IS BULIMIA NERVOSA DANGEROUS?

Without treatment, bulimia nervosa is a chronic condition. People struggling with bulimia nervosa are likely to experience many health problems, including dental erosion, periodontal disease, gastrointestinal distress and discomfort, swollen salivary glands, sensitivity to cold, anemia, dehydration, and constipation. More severe and potentially fatal effects include esophageal damage, osteoporosis, electrolyte imbalance, and cardiac arrest. Bulimia nervosa also is associated with increased rates of depression, anxiety disorders, alcoholism and

(cont.)

substance abuse, and suicide. Eating disorders commonly lead to problems in intimate relationships, friendships, employment, and parenting.

HOW DOES BEHAVIOR AND THINKING AFFECT BULIMIA NERVOSA?

The cognitive-behavioral theory of bulimia nervosa suggests that an individual defines and evaluates her/himself excessively in terms of shape and weight. The pursuit of thinness and/or maintaining weight loss is the main focus for the individual with an eating disorder. The tendency to judge self-worth in terms of weight drives the individual to diet restrictively. Strict dieting, in turn, leads to psychological deprivation and physiological hunger. When combined with life stress, negative emotions, and poor self-image, hunger can trigger a binge. A binge elicits feelings of guilt, shame, and self-loathing and uncomfortable feelings of fullness. To compensate for the binge and a fear of gaining weight, an individual with bulimia nervosa may vomit, use laxatives, abuse diuretics, exercise excessively, or restrict food intake. The continuation of strict dieting and self-critical thinking propels the binge cycle. The belief that through weight control one can increase self-esteem leads to the exact opposite—psychological distress, guilt, shame, and worthlessness.

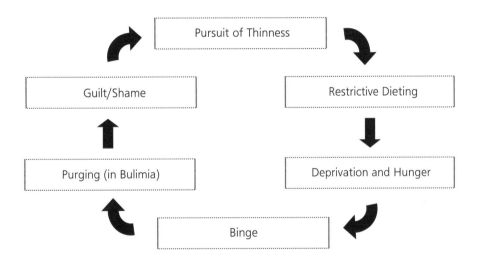

WHAT IS COGNITIVE-BEHAVIORAL TREATMENT?

Cognitive-behavioral therapy is a short-term, skills-based treatment that focuses on the behaviors, thoughts, and coping skills that contribute to and maintain your eating disorder. Multiple research studies have found cognitive-behavioral therapy to be a superior form of treatment for bulimia nervosa. It is more effective than a variety of other therapies and is regarded as the first line of treatment for eating disorders. Cognitive-behavioral therapy addresses the psychological, familial, and societal factors associated with eating disorders and is centered on the principle that there are both behavioral and attitudinal disturbances in eating, weight, and shape. Cognitive-behavioral therapy directly targets the binge cycle. You will work together with your therapist to change eating behaviors, to discontinue purging, and to challenge rules that prevent natural and healthy eating patterns. Adoption of more flexible eating patterns and learning new coping skills are central to preventing binges. Treatment also targets the thoughts and feelings that can trigger binge eating, including perfectionism and "all-or-nothing" thinking. By identifying the biases in your thinking, challenging your negative thoughts, learning new stress and emotion coping skills, and relearning moderate, healthy eating, you have a good chance of

(cont.)

getting over your eating disorder. Cognitive-behavioral treatment also works to improve your body image. The final phase of treatment is relapse prevention, where you will work with your therapist to develop and practice strategies to maintain your progress and to prevent a relapse to bingeing, purging, and unhealthy eating habits. The skills learned throughout treatment will help you maintain your progress on your own after treatment ends.

ARE MEDICATIONS USEFUL?

Medications alone are unlikely to help your eating disorder. Some research suggests that certain antidepressant medications, when combined with cognitive-behavioral treatment, may improve bingeing and depression. If you are experiencing severe anxiety or depression in addition to your eating disorder, medications may help you get more out of your treatment. Your therapist will discuss whether medications are a good option for you.

WHAT IS EXPECTED OF YOU AS A PATIENT?

Cognitive-behavioral treatment for bulimia nervosa initially may be anxiety provoking, yet you are likely to feel more comfortable once you observe how quickly treatment disrupts the binge cycle. As a patient, you will be asked to give the therapy an honest try and to practice skills learned between sessions. Homework, regular attendance, and honesty with your therapist are crucial for your treatment to be effective.

FORM 3.2. Case Conceptualization Worksheet

Instructions: This worksheet is to be completed by the therapist, typically between the intake assessment and first treatment session. It should include all relevant cognitions, behaviors, and symptoms identified through the Evaluation of Eating Disorders form, other intake assessment measures, and the patient's description of presenting problems.

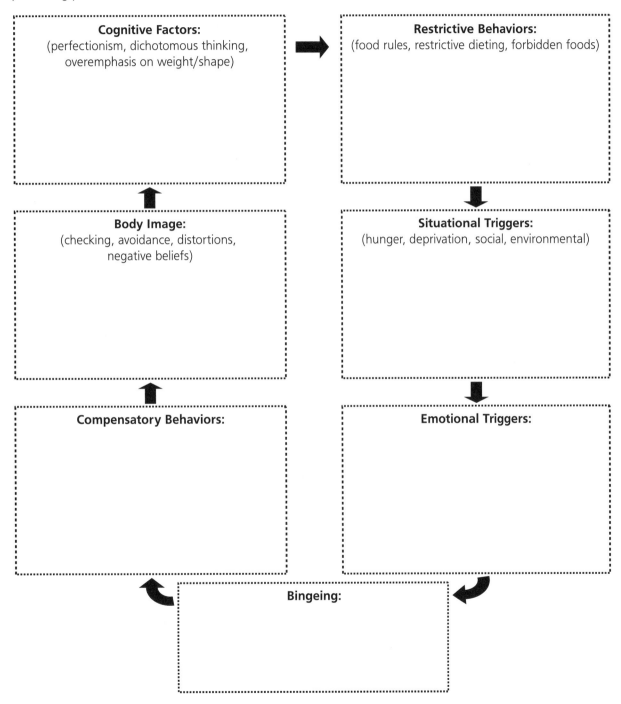

Cognitive Factors:
(perfectionism, dichotomous thinking, overemphasis on weight/shape)

Restrictive Behaviors:
(food rules, restrictive dieting, forbidden foods)

Body Image:
(checking, avoidance, distortions, negative beliefs)

Situational Triggers:
(hunger, deprivation, social, environmental)

Compensatory Behaviors:

Emotional Triggers:

Bingeing:

CHAPTER 4

Detailed Treatment Plan for Bulimia Nervosa

CBT for BN is traditionally delivered in 20 outpatient psychotherapy sessions over the course of 6 months. All treatment will follow the same basic cognitive-behavioral model, although specific cognitive-behavioral interventions will be tailored to each patient based on eating disorder severity, presenting symptoms, and the therapist's case formulation. Treatment sessions are typically held weekly. In some instances, it can be useful to hold twice-weekly sessions in order to increase early symptom improvement and to bolster motivation. This may be particularly useful for patients with more severe symptoms, lower motivation for treatment, or a history of low treatment compliance. Treatment may last more than 6 months if additional treatment is warranted to address comorbid conditions (e.g., depression), to allow adequate time to respond to any treatment setbacks or resistance, or to improve functioning in other life areas (e.g., social engagement).

The basic **structure of each 50-minute treatment session** is to set a collaborative agenda with the patient, thoroughly review the past week's homework, introduce and practice one or two cognitive-behavioral interventions, assign homework for the coming week, and end by summarizing the session. During each session the therapist and patient can also address roadblocks and difficulties encountered in carrying out self-help assignments. The application of many of the cognitive-behavioral techniques is summarized in the following section.

SOCIALIZATION TO TREATMENT

In the first session, after the initial assessment is completed and a case formulation has been made, it is important to educate patients about the cognitive-behavioral theory of BN. Patients may be given a copy of Form 3.1, Information for Patients about Bulimia Nervosa, at their intake session or the following treatment session. This handout contains a description of the cognitive-behavioral model of BN. A discussion of this model can demonstrate to patients how their excessive focus on shape and weight creates dissatisfaction and drives increasingly rigid attempts to control their diet. Dieting, in turn, leads to feelings of deprivation and hunger, both of which have been shown to trigger bingeing. Because bingeing results in feelings of shame and discomfort, patients have learned to purge to alleviate their psychological and physical symptoms. Purging and bingeing are both temporarily reinforcing as they initially reduce negative affect. However, both behaviors ultimately result in additional negative affect, shame, and self-critical thoughts. After a binge–purge episode, patients then typically vow to "try harder" and "be more disciplined" the following day, continuing the rigid, restrictive cycle. It should be explained to patients that each of these symptoms will need to be targeted to fully disrupt their eating disorder, and that they will learn new strategies to manage these symptoms throughout treatment (see Figure 2.1). Patients typically feel relieved and hopeful after discussing this cycle. They feel understood by their therapist and more confident that treatment can help.

Setting treatment goals is a logical next step, one that will also occur in **session 1.** Patients should be encouraged to define their own treatment goals, and the therapist should assist as needed to model the collaborative nature of the therapeutic relationship. Suggested treatment goals include discontinuing bingeing and purging, attaining a healthy body weight, improving body image, improving mood, resuming normal activities, and improving interpersonal relationships. Regardless of patients' body weight at treatment intake, weight loss cannot be a goal of treatment as dietary restriction is likely to maintain binge eating. If patients are at a low body weight at the start of treatment, some weight gain is likely upon resuming regular meal intake. For patients who begin treatment overweight, weight loss may or may not occur once bingeing is discontinued. If weight loss is a reasonable goal for the patient, weight management interventions can be introduced upon completion of the 20-session treatment plan, assuming bingeing has ceased and food intake has stabilized.

Therapists should then provide patients with a good understanding of the treatment process. To help prevent early attrition, patients ought to have a full understanding of the expected length of treatment, the use of homework, and the likelihood of setbacks along the way. Patients should be encouraged to discuss any concerns or waning motivation with their therapist as treatment progresses. Strategies for effectively managing patient resistance, setbacks, and low motivation are discussed in the section Possible "Roadblocks" and Treatment Resistance, later in this chapter.

MOTIVATION

It is normal for patients to feel ambivalent about change at the outset of treatment, and interventions to increase motivation can improve treatment retention and engagement. Motivational enhancement interventions will be used in **sessions 1 and 2,** and again later in treatment if warranted. It is most useful if therapists adopt a nondirective and nonconfrontational stance while eliciting from patients the potential **advantages and disadvantages of change.** Toward this end, the Motivation Worksheet (Form 4.1) is a useful tool to help patients identify and record the pros and cons of their eating disorder behaviors. Therapists may wish to complete the Motivation Worksheet together with patients in session or to assign this as homework. Patients should be encouraged to consider the medical, social, occupational, familial, and psychological consequences already experienced as a result of their eating disorder as well as potential future consequences. Likewise, the current and future expected advantages of the eating disorder should be fully discussed. Patients should be asked to consider whether the eating disorder is in line with their long-term goals. This may include consideration of how bingeing, purging, overemphasis on body shape, and dietary restriction affect mood, anxiety, self-esteem, social functioning, time and energy, and occupational responsibilities. Patients often report feeling motivated for change, and can list a variety of advantages to being free of their eating disorder:

- They will not binge and purge.
- They will no longer be obsessed with food.
- They can eat socially again.
- They won't feel controlled by food and restriction.
- They will no longer feel ashamed.
- They won't have to hide their eating disorder anymore.
- They can be a good role model for their children.
- They can gain back the trust of loved ones.
- They can resume currently restricted physical activities.
- They will develop healthier coping strategies.
- They can develop a normal relationship with food.

Of course, patients will also be able to cite disadvantages of change:

- Weight gain
- Increased anxiety
- Fear of the unknown
- Fear of losing control
- Possibility of failing
- No longer using food to cope
- Losing one's "friend"

Patients often need to return to this worksheet throughout treatment whenever their motivation begins to wane.

BEHAVIORAL CHANGE

The goal of the first phase of treatment, which comprises sessions 2–7, is to help clients discontinue problematic behaviors while adopting more healthful, less rigid eating and coping behaviors.

Food Records

The most critical component of behavioral change is the Food Record (Form 4.2), the daily monitoring form used to identify the patient's food intake patterns, to determine binge triggers, and to raise awareness of emotional and cognitive factors. The Food Record form will be introduced to patients in **session 2** and will be utilized throughout treatment. It is imperative that patients complete the Food Record as close to the time of eating as possible to ensure accurate recording of all food intake, portion sizes, and any situational or emotional triggers. Patients should be instructed to record all food and drink consumed, including diet soda, teas, and other beverages. There is space for them to record the time they ate, the specific location, the general quantity consumed, whether it constituted a binge (denoted by *), whether they used laxatives or vomited afterward (denoted by V/L), and any additional comments. A binge is defined as consuming an objectively large amount of food in a short period of time while feeling out of control. It is useful to share this definition with patients. Smaller quantities ingested or periods of prolonged "grazing" may feel uncomfortable for patients and thus should be noted in the comments column. These "subjective binges" are not true binges; however, they do provide valuable information about patients' food rules and consumption patterns. The comments column is also useful for patients to indicate their hunger and satiety levels, satisfaction with foods consumed, urges to binge, specific interpersonal and situational binge triggers, and awareness of strong emotions throughout the day. It is important that patients not count calories or try to stay within a certain daily caloric limit as dietary restriction perpetuates obsessive thinking and can trigger binge episodes. Therapists should watch for indications of this behavior. Patients often feel ashamed about recording large quantities of food ingested, and thus may stop recording when a binge occurs. Therapists should address this problem proactively by encouraging patients to record all food intake, emphasizing that accurately reporting binge foods ingested is the best way to identify triggers and to ultimately disrupt the bingeing.

When introducing the use of food records to the patient, it is often helpful to complete one together in session by reviewing what the patient ate thus far that day or during the previous day. A sample completed record can also be provided for the patient's reference (see Figure 4.1). The first week that food records are assigned, the patient should be asked to monitor without changing her food intake to allow the therapist and patient to assess her typical patterns. After the initial week of assigned food records, the therapist should dedicate a significant portion of session time to reviewing completed records. This underscores the importance of food records, allows the patient to explain her notations, and enables the therapist and patient to begin noting restriction–binge–purge patterns. The patient will continue to keep food records throughout the remainder of treatment, and the therapist and patient will briefly review completed records at the start of each session. The therapist can keep all completed food records in the patient's file so that they are readily available to review in subsequent sessions. The patient will often find it useful to look over old food records to note treatment progress, to obtain evidence for cognitive restructuring exercises, and to identify long-standing food intake patterns. The food records also will be utilized in later weeks to note the patient's use of alternative behavioral strategies, to identify food-related cognitions and emotions, and to record successful resistance of urges.

Patients often resist completing food records, citing fears that paying additional attention to food intake will lead to even more obsessive thoughts about food. Patients also typically fear that food records will lead to more frequent bingeing. Although most patients fear these outcomes, they rarely occur. If patients are not convinced by discussion alone, the food records can be framed as a 2-week experiment. If patients still find them difficult or uncomfortable after a 2-week trial, the assignment can be revisited. Practical problems with completion may also be raised, such as how to complete records while out to dinner or while at work. It is important to address patients' fears up front and to problem solve any expected or actual difficulties with completion. Patients have found it useful to carry the food records folded in their handbag or pocket so they are always accessible. Many patients also put a Post-it Note on their refrigerator to

Day: M (T) W Th F Sa Su

Date: _November 30_____

Time	Location	Food/Drink Consumed	*	V/L	Emotions/Triggers/ Urges/Satisfaction
7:30	Home— kitchen table	Bowl of blueberries Coffee w/ Splenda			Today is going to be a stressful day! Good, healthy breakfast
10 am	Desk	Coffee w/ Splenda			
1:15 pm	Desk	Small tossed mixed greens with chicken, cucumbers, tomatoes, & broccoli			Good lunch. Very full.
3:15	Desk	Seltzer—1 can			
5 pm	Conference room	Diet Coke			Tired. Irritable. Stressed.
7:30 pm	Desk	5 Peanut M&Ms			In stressful meeting. Couldn't resist. Feel so guilty. Should've waited until dinner.
8:45 pm	Desk	Sushi—4 pieces & 1 roll			So busy with work, barely noticed eating. Will be a late night :(
9 pm	Desk	Handful M&Ms	*		Boss just criticized my work. Angry. Lonely. Tired.
		Package peanut butter crackers	*		Already blown it. Feel so fat. Shouldn't have eaten those M&Ms.
		Package Oreo cookies	*		
		3 more Oreos	*		
		2 handfuls mixed nuts	*		
		5 mini Reese's cups	*		
		2 chocolate donuts	*	V	Relief to vomit. I am a disgusting pig.

FIGURE 4.1. Example of a Completed Food Record.

serve as a reminder until recording becomes a habit. For public situations in which it is difficult to record, patients have problem solved by completing the sheets in the bathroom or jotting notes on a napkin to later transfer to their food record. Patients are typically motivated to fully comply if the therapist explains how food records predict treatment success. In addition, it is useful to explain to patients that although their concerns and fears are completely normal, they have proved unfounded with many prior patients. Many recovered patients have spontaneously commented at the end of their treatment that they were initially quite skeptical of food records but now recognize how critically important they were in the treatment process.

Weekly Weighing

Also in the first session following intake (**session 2**), the therapist should introduce in-session weekly weighing. Patients with BN tend to either weigh themselves multiple times daily in an obsessive manner or to avoid the scale altogether. Weekly weighing is used to counteract these extreme tendencies while obtaining important feedback about any body weight changes. Weekly weighing allows patients to habituate to this feared stimulus. As weight fluctuates daily (even hourly) depending on food and liquid intake, salt intake, hormone levels, weather, and other factors, no useful information is obtained by weighing more often than once weekly. In fact, many patients recognize that weighing themselves too frequently only serves to keep them overly focused on their shape and weight, and the number on the scale disproportionately determines their daily mood. Likewise, avoidance of the scale maintains the fear of the number, and does not allow patients to disconfirm any of their food- and weight-related fears. Often patients are concerned about being weighed by the therapist or do not want to see the number themselves. The therapist can reduce this common fear by introducing weekly weighing in a straightforward, matter-of-fact manner. In the same way that a doctor must assess one's blood pressure as part of an annual physical examination, weekly weighing must be completed to stay on top of any changes in therapy. In all the remaining treatment sessions, weekly weighing will be done at the start of the session along with the check-in, agenda setting, and food records review.

Calculating Body Mass Index

After the initial weigh-in, the therapist and patient should together calculate the patient's BMI (see Form B.6 in Appendix B). This may happen in either **session 1 or 2,** depending on when the first body weight is taken. BMI is simply a standardized reference for body weight that takes height into account. Although it is not a perfect measure, it is a useful tool to categorize a patient as underweight, normal weight, or overweight. It is important to give this feedback to the patient, showing her the BMI handout to help put into perspective her actual body size. Patients with eating disorders, especially those who are underweight or low-normal weight, often see themselves in a distorted way. This is an opportune moment to reiterate the importance of a nondiet approach in this treatment. Patients should be given the feedback that they are unlikely to see any dramatic changes (losses or gains) in body weight over the course of treatment despite making significant changes in their eating patterns. An exception, of course, is that underweight patients will be expected to increase their food intake over the course of treatment, and regaining to a normal body weight may be an explicit treatment goal.

Discontinuing All Compensatory Behaviors

Early in treatment, typically during **session 3,** the therapist should work with patients to discontinue all compensatory behaviors. Compensatory behaviors are defined as any attempt to offset the effects of overeating to prevent weight gain. Patients often describe their compensatory behaviors as a form of self-punishment following bingeing. Vomiting is the most commonly used compensatory behavior by patients with BN, although they may also try laxative use, diuretic use, enemas, excessive exercise, or periods of fasting. Ideally, compensatory behaviors, including vomiting and laxative use, should be ceased immediately. Purging maintains the binge cycle by giving patients an illusion of control over weight gain, thereby effectively giving permission for future binges. It is, therefore, important that this part of the cycle be disrupted as quickly as possible. While discussing immediate cessation with patients, it is important to emphasize the ineffectiveness of using purging and laxatives to prevent weight gain. (Form 4.3, Information for Patients about Purging, is a useful educational overview that the therapist can distribute to supplement in-session discussions.) Laxatives do not at all prevent the absorption of calories, because they operate after food has been digested. Any noticeable weight loss after laxative use is due to water loss, which will be regained immediately. Vomiting following binges will prevent the absorption of some ingested calories, although it is much less effective in this regard than patients realize (Kaye, Weltzin, Hsu, McConaha, & Bolton, 1993). Vomiting has significant medical and emotional costs for patients, and these should be elicited and thoroughly discussed. Vomiting is a dangerous behavior and is directly responsible for nearly all of the medical and dental complications associated with BN. Recurrent vomiting can cause dehydration and electrolyte imbalance, which in turn are responsible for constipation, kidney failure, slowed pulse, low blood pressure, irregular heartbeat, cardiac distress, and metabolic alkalosis. The regurgitation of stomach acid while vomiting contributes to dental decay, swollen salivary glands, mouth ulcers, irritable bowel syndrome, ulcers, sore throat, damage to the esophagus, and gastrointestinal bleeding. Patients often disclose feeling shame and disgust and may limit their social engagements as a result of their vomiting behaviors. They may also recognize the role vomiting plays in permitting larger and more frequent binges because of the false reassurance that the binge can be "gotten rid of." In addition to the aforementioned consequences, repeated laxative use can result in dehydration, bowel damage, and long-term severe constipation.

Most patients are able to discontinue compensatory behaviors immediately, and this approach is optimal. Therapists should ask patients to commit to a week without vomiting or laxative use, even if they should binge. This can be framed as an experiment to test how long the discomfort and urges last following a binge. The therapist can ask patients for a specific set of predictions regarding how long the urge to purge or the feeling of discomfort will last. These urges typically subside rapidly. By recognizing the ephemeral nature of discomfort associated with these urges, patients will begin to see that purging is a harmful and unnecessary solution to a problem that is only temporary.

As already mentioned, vomiting and laxative use are ineffective means to prevent weight gain following binges, and thus discontinuation of purging behaviors rarely results in weight gain. A patient who has been abusing laxatives may experience temporary bloating and constipation upon discontinuation of laxatives, and this artificial weight gain typically lasts several days to several weeks. These points should be emphasized because patients may be reluctant to discontinue purging for fear of gaining weight. It also should be emphasized that most patients report bingeing less frequently (and without any concerted effort to do so) soon after they discontinue purging.

Patients may find it useful to **identify alternative behaviors** (e.g., brush teeth, clean toilet, write in journal) or **coping statements** (e.g., "I will not purge because I want to get better") to get themselves through urges to purge following a binge. Patients may also find it useful to review the information in Form 4.3 while experiencing an urge to purge. Patients should be instructed to record their urges to purge on their food records, including any successful resistance to purging.

At the next session, patients' efforts to discontinue purging should be reviewed carefully. Any attempts to resist purging should be reinforced, and successful resistance should be analyzed to identify what made this possible. The therapist also should elicit patients' reactions whenever they did not purge after a binge. For all instances of bingeing without purging, the duration of bloating and discomfort should be assessed. Patients often recognize that the discomfort did not last as long as predicted and that they felt less guilty in the absence of purging.

Delaying Purging

If the patient continued to purge throughout the week despite significant efforts to abstain, the therapist should instead recommend delayed purging. Delaying purging following a binge serves as incremental exposure and response prevention for the patient, similar to the interventions used in CBT for obsessive–compulsive disorder. Delaying the purging behaviors disrupts the learned association between the stimulus (bingeing) and the compulsive response (purging), thereby weakening the reinforcing effect of the purging. The patient should wait a specified period of time (e.g., 10 minutes) after a binge before she engages in her usual purging behaviors. During that time period, the patient should do nothing but sit with her anxiety and discomfort. If the desire to purge remains following the elapsed time, the patient may then purge. If the urge to purge has passed, as often happens, then she should not purge. After each instance of delayed purging, the waiting period should be lengthened (e.g., to 20 minutes), and this sequence should be repeated as often as necessary to achieve complete abstinence from purging. It should be noted that delayed purging is typically used for vomiting behaviors, although it can be applied to laxative use if longer waiting periods are utilized.

Regular Eating

Also in **session 3,** the therapist will help the patient to adopt a regular, planned eating pattern. Initiating regular, planned meals and snacks to be eaten throughout the day helps disrupt the periods of deprivation and restriction that are common in BN and that are a central trigger for binge episodes. Returning to the cognitive-behavioral model, the rationale should be carefully explained to the patient, including the ways in which deprivation drives the eating disorder and how dietary restriction controls the patient rather than giving her control over her environment (e.g., avoidance, social disruption, obsession with food).

The patient should be instructed to **eat every 3–4 hours** throughout the day, regardless of hunger, and **to not eat between these scheduled times.** A sample planned eating schedule is outlined in Figure 4.2. It must be emphasized that the included sample schedule is not intended to

```
┌─────────────────────────────────────────┐
│            A Sample Schedule            │
│                                         │
│   7:00 A.M.      Wake                   │
│                                         │
│   7:30 A.M.      Breakfast              │
│                                         │
│   10:30 A.M.     Morning snack          │
│                                         │
│   1:00 P.M.      Lunch                  │
│                                         │
│   4:00 P.M.      Afternoon snack        │
│                                         │
│   7:30 P.M.      Dinner                 │
│                                         │
│   10:30 P.M.     Evening snack          │
│                                         │
│   11:30 P.M.     Bedtime                │
└─────────────────────────────────────────┘
```

FIGURE 4.2. Regular planned eating.

be a prescription, and there will be significant variability in eating schedules among patients and across days. Eating on schedule must be made a priority by the patient and will often necessitate planning ahead. Although the patient will not be actively dieting, it should be emphasized that what she eats now is less important than the timing of her eating. Eating on schedule and keeping daily food records is the priority at this phase and will serve as the foundation for upcoming treatment interventions.

Within an hour of waking, the patient should consume her first meal. The remainder of the day's meal and snack times can then be set, scheduled at 3- to 4-hour intervals. The day's schedule can be noted at the top of the food record, and any potential difficulties (e.g., lunch meeting at work) can be problem solved in advance. With this schedule, the patient will need to consume approximately three meals and two to three snacks daily, which is often much more than her typical intake. The patient should be reminded that this increased intake is what will help prevent bingeing. Although the patient will typically fear weight gain, this is unlikely because the caloric intake from more regular eating is offset by a lack of bingeing. Eating every 3–4 hours throughout the day prevents the extreme hunger and deprivation that can trigger bingeing, it breaks some of the patient's problematic "food rules," and it helps reset the patient's hunger and satiety signals. Because the patient must not eat between scheduled times, regular eating offers **practice in resisting urges** for shorter periods of time. When faced with a tempting situation or trigger food, for example, the patient may find it useful to remind herself that she needs to wait only 45 minutes before the next scheduled time to eat.

Functional Analysis of Binge Triggers

Binge frequency is often reduced by the fourth treatment session as a result of the use of food records, regular eating, and discontinued purging. Patients, however, are usually eager to cease bingeing altogether. Binges most often occur when there is access to a trigger food, when patients are alone and without a schedule, and following a momentary urge. Trigger foods include those foods about which patients have "food rules," that they consider "bad" and restricted, and that they rarely consume outside of a binge episode (e.g., potato chips, cakes, cookies, full-fat ice cream, chocolate candy, cheese). In addition, patients report feeling "numb," secretive, and disconnected during a binge, while they may report strong negative emotions prior to the binge. The therapist will regularly review food records with patients to determine which situations, people, emotions, and food are particularly likely to precede a binge episode. Binge triggers that occurred prior to starting therapy can also be studied from memory. The functional analysis of past triggers to determine those times when patients are most vulnerable is an important component of treatment. Functional analysis typically occurs starting in **session 4** and will continue throughout treatment. After patients' idiosyncratic binge triggers are identified through functional analysis, interventions to plan for and prevent bingeing can be targeted to those areas.

Stimulus Control

At approximately **session 4,** the therapist introduces patients to stimulus control techniques, outlined in Form 4.4. Stimulus control techniques are behavioral strategies that help structure patients' environments and decrease access to trigger foods, thereby preventing bingeing. To avoid bingeing, patients should intentionally limit their *access* to trigger foods by keeping those foods out of their homes and workplaces whenever possible. When this is not possible, trigger foods should be made less accessible (e.g., back of cabinet, in freezer) to help prevent urges and to create a delay between urge and action. In addition, patients find it helpful to have alternate, safer foods readily *available* for snacking and meals. If patients are feeling particularly vulnerable to bingeing on a given day, places and situations that include binge foods should also be avoided (e.g., not going to the grocery store after work, selecting a safe restaurant to meet a friend).

Planning ahead, including scheduling the times and content of meals and snacks, is crucial to prevent binges. This is especially important for holidays, special events, and busy days, when trigger foods may be present and willpower lower. When eating any meal or snack, it is helpful for patients to *serve the portion* they intend to eat and put the rest away. Keeping the meal off the table, storing leftovers in the freezer, or throwing away any extra food are all good strategies to prevent overeating, which can be the beginning of a binge. The saying "Out of sight, out of mind" applies here. If food is not visible or available, patients are less likely to experience urges to binge. Creating a set *routine* for meals and snacks helps break any old associations between eating and other activities. When eating, patients should give their full attention to their food. They should not watch television, use the computer, or read while eating. All meals and snacks should be eaten in the same location within the home and while sitting. After developing a set routine around eating, patients will be less likely to experience urges to binge while watching television, at the movies, or in certain rooms of their home. While eating, patients should also concentrate on eating *slowly* and *mindfully*, noticing the textures and flavors in their foods. Mindfulness refers to the act of bringing one's full awareness to the present moment and, when applied to eating, means bringing full attention to the experience of consuming a food or beverage. When patients eat in this way, they are more likely to feel satisfied and full, and thus less likely to go on to binge. To signal the end of a meal or snack, patients should *write down* all food and drink consumed and then *move* out of the dining location. This combination of recording and moving reduces the likelihood of continued mindless eating. Whenever patients have the desire to eat unplanned foods, they should utilize the *5-minute rule,* which requires them to wait 5 minutes before giving in to any urges. During those 5 minutes, patients may distract themselves with another activity. More often than not, this pause allows the urge to pass and gives patients the opportunity to reconsider whether or not they want to binge.

Urge Surfing

Although stimulus control techniques will reduce the frequency of urges to binge, not all situations can be carefully controlled. When urges to binge do arise spontaneously, the patient will need to have a plan to ride out these urges to avoid bingeing. The patient should be encouraged to watch her urges to notice their duration and intensity. Most urges last less than 10 minutes, and if the patient can wait out that period, the urge will pass and bingeing will not occur. One strategy for riding out urges is "urge surfing," a technique adapted from CBT for addictions (Marlatt & Witkiewitz, 2005). Urge surfing can be introduced and practiced in **session 5.** For this exercise, the patient imagines riding the urge like an ocean wave. The premise of urge surfing is to watch rather than act on or struggle against the natural pattern of all behavioral urges. Urges arise suddenly, gain power as they approach, peak gradually, and then subside relatively quickly. Just as with a wave, if the patient struggles with the urge and tries to stand tall against it, the urge will knock her down. If, on the other hand, the patient lets the urge come and go without acting on it, the ride will be smooth. This imaginal exercise can be introduced and practiced in session, and the patient should then practice using this coping strategy on her own between sessions.

A common problem with urge surfing is when the patient reports that urges seem to last much longer than 10 minutes, with some urges lasting all day. It should be explained to the patient that this is likely a series of individual urges rather than a single, prolonged urge. The patient can, therefore, ride out each individual urge and notice the breaks between urges rather than feel overwhelmed by one seemingly never-ending urge. In addition, urges that repeatedly arise may be due to the presence of a specific trigger (e.g., binge food readily available, interpersonal trigger), which should then be addressed using stimulus control strategies to prevent further urges.

Alternative Activities

Another useful strategy for getting through urges is to use alternative activities, which are most helpful when identified in advance. This strategy should be introduced to the patient in **session 5.** The therapist and patient will start by consulting the functional analysis of binge triggers conducted in the previous session. Common binge triggers include hunger, strong negative or positive emotion, overeating, breaking a food rule, alcohol, social situations, anxiety, and loneliness. For each previously identified binge trigger, the therapist and patient can brainstorm alternative, non-food activities to replace bingeing, using Form 4.5. For example, a patient who is tempted to binge when bored may instead decide to read a novel, clean a closet, play a game, or do a yoga DVD. Engaging in another activity distracts the patient long enough for the urge to pass, and the more often a patient successfully averts a binge, the more confidence she builds to ride out future urges. It is recommended that the patient write down her chosen alternative behaviors and then carry the list in a wallet or handbag to serve as a reminder of possible alternative urge coping strategies in the moment. In addition, the patient can consult the Checklist of Possible Alternative Coping Strategies (see Form 4.6) for other coping options.

Problem Solving and Planning Ahead

In addition to planning alternative strategies to manage past binge triggers, which are likely to recur, patients will benefit from planning ahead for upcoming difficult situations. Often patients know in advance that a situation will be difficult and will likely result in the urge to binge. Common situational triggers include social events (e.g., a party, a barbecue, dining out with friends), a stressful work situation, a weekend with no social plans, and travel. Patients often report feeling anticipatory anxiety, hopelessness, or a strong desire to avoid these situations because they view bingeing as inevitable. The goal of this intervention is to help patients regain confidence about these potential trigger situations, and to help them identify specific behaviors and thoughts that will help them get through these situations without bingeing.

Beginning in **session 6,** the therapist will introduce the three steps to problem solving:

1. Identify that an upcoming situation may trigger bingeing.
2. Plan ahead for how to effectively manage this situation without bingeing.
3. After the situation has passed, review whether the plan was effective in preventing bingeing.

The second step of problem solving will occur in session, with the therapist and the patient together identifying alternative ways to approach the situation without bingeing. This second step involves brainstorming and selecting specific, healthier behaviors and thoughts for use before, during, and after the situation. For example, the patient may report feeling vulnerable to bingeing during the coming weekend because she will be going out on a first date. From prior experience, the patient knows she is quite likely to feel anxious in anticipation of and during the date, and is likely to feel self-critical afterward. The patient fears that after the date she will ruminate about all the embarrassing things she said, convince herself that she "blew it," and dwell on how she will be single forever. She will then want to binge because she feels alone, hopeless, and depressed. To prevent bingeing, the therapist and patient create a plan for her following the date. First, the patient will change her clothes and brush her teeth. This signals that her day is ending and she will not eat again. The patient will then make a list of everything that went well on the date to help counteract her tendency to ruminate on the negative. Last, the patient will go to bed. She will remind herself that this is important because she is tired, and she will only feel worse if she stays up and binges.

The third and final step of problem solving is critical, and this involves reviewing whether the plan was effective in preventing bingeing. It is important to note whether the patient followed the plan and, if not, what prevented her from doing so. The patient should also be asked to describe any strategies that did not help prevent bingeing and what may have worked better in the situation. This is an opportunity for the patient to learn from both her successes and her mistakes and to then be better equipped to prepare for future scenarios.

The patient should be encouraged to discuss any potentially difficult situations with the therapist in advance so that problem solving can be practiced throughout the remainder of treatment.

Relaxation Training

Deficits in coping skills are assumed to be one reason why patients with BN binge when confronted with strong, negative emotion. Bingeing is viewed as a dysfunctional emotional coping strategy. Thus, patients will greatly benefit from learning new, healthier coping strategies. While other emotion regulation skills will be introduced later in treatment, the therapist can teach patients relaxation training during **session 6.** Diaphragmatic breathing is one form of relaxation training (Kabat-Zinn, 1990; Wilson, 1996). The following narrative will allow the therapist to demonstrate diaphragmatic breathing in session and for patients to practice on their own between sessions. As little as 5–10 minutes of in-session training will adequately demonstrate this skill to patients and allow them to begin a daily at-home practice.

> "To practice deep breathing, simply sit comfortably with your legs uncrossed, your hands in your lap or at your sides. Let your head fall back and, if you feel comfortable, close your eyes. You may also fix your eyes on one point in the room. Take several breaths as normal. Now direct your attention to your breath, noticing the sensations as you inhale and as you exhale. If you find that your mind wanders during this exercise, simply redirect your attention back to your breath. Now place one hand on your abdomen, just below your rib cage. This hand should rise and fall with each breath. Breathe in slowly through your nose, allowing the air to travel deep into your body, then circling back out slowly, exhaling from your mouth. With each breath, concentrate on breathing more slowly and more deeply. You may intentionally push out your abdomen to make more room for your breath. Breathe in slowly, counting to 5. Inhaling for 1-2-3-4-5. Now slowly exhale, also counting to 5. Exhaling for 1-2-3-4-5. Continue breathing deeply, counting along with your breath. Breathe in for 1-2-3-4-5. Breathe out for 1-2-3-4-5. There is no right or wrong way to breathe, simply try to keep your mind focused on your breath. Try to make each breath slower and deeper than the last. You might imagine breathing in fresh, clean air each time you inhale and, as you exhale, breathing out any tension or stress. Without judgment, notice any tension or discomfort in your body. Allow your breath to relax your body and your mind. Continue to slowly breathe in and out. Breathe in for 1-2-3-4-5. Breathe out for 1-2-3-4-5. Take several more slow, deep breaths, still keeping your mind focused on your breathing. Now, when you are ready, you may open your eyes."

The therapist may wish to record this in-session training to allow patients to repeat this deep-breathing exercise on their own between sessions. Alternatively, patients may practice deep breathing at home by using these written instructions (see Form 4.7), a meditation MP3 file or application, or a commercial CD. The patients' homework for the coming week should be to practice deep-breathing exercises twice daily for approximately 10 minutes each. With daily practice, patients will learn to better cope with stress, negative affect, and urges to binge.

Reviewing Treatment Progress

Each treatment session should begin with a 5-minute review of the prior week's homework and a check-in about any happenings from the previous week. This is an excellent opportunity for the patient and therapist to regularly highlight any treatment progress to date. It is useful to review both effective and ineffective strategies, binge–purge frequency, and adherence to planned eating. The therapist and patient should together problem solve any difficulties implementing new skills, any treatment setbacks, and any concerning weight changes. While reviewing food records at each session, the therapist should notice the quantity of food consumed at meals and snacks, particularly if the patient presents as underweight. As the patient becomes more comfortable eating on schedule, the therapist may give the patient feedback on her food intake, encouraging her to eat "normal" portions. The patient may benefit from observing how much others eat and using these observations to better gauge her own portion sizes. The therapist should also address any noticeable caloric restriction or avoidance of particular foods. To help maintain motivation for change, the patient should be encouraged to notice and verbalize her own improvement.

Although the therapist and patient will review treatment progress and assess homework completion at the start of each treatment session, a more formal and extensive review is warranted during **session 7.** This session marks the end of the first phase of treatment (the behavioral interventions), and the patient will likely have made significant progress by this point. At this stage, it is common for the patient to note that she feels less obsessed with food, is more relaxed when eating with others, is relieved that she no longer binges and purges (or does so less frequently), is less moody, and is somewhat less obsessed with weight. The patient may also have experienced one or more significant setbacks to date, which can be discussed and problem solved if necessary. Treatment has also progressed enough to allow the patient to evaluate her initial fears about treatment or specific treatment interventions. By reviewing her progress to date, any change in body weight, and current eating patterns, the patient can evaluate whether there was merit to early concerns about weight gain or an increased obsession with food.

COGNITIVE RESTRUCTURING

The second phase of treatment, beginning at approximately **session 8,** is focused on identifying and adapting the patient's problematic thought patterns. This phase helps disrupt the cycle of overattention to body shape and weight, rigid standards for the self, and extreme adherence to food rules. Cognitive restructuring is a key component of CBT because it reinforces and helps maintain the behavioral changes made and frees the patient from her overemphasis on body shape. Attempts to interrupt problematic behaviors up to this point in treatment have likely provided clues about the patient's negative thought patterns, existing food rules, and distorted body image beliefs. Comprehensive reviews of cognitive therapy can be found in *Cognitive Behavior Therapy: Basics and Beyond* (Beck, 2011), and *Cognitive Therapy Techniques: A Practitioner's Guide* (Leahy, 2003).

The Thought–Behavior Connection

To help the patient better understand the role of cognitions in her eating disorder, the therapist should explain the thought–behavior connection, which is the way in which automatic thoughts influence one's behavioral and emotional reactions to situations. All situations include some element of ambiguity that requires interpretation, which is why different people may interpret the same situation very differently. We cannot, for example, know the future consequences of an event or what others are thinking. Depending on our belief system and prior experiences, we insert judgment into the situations we experience. While subjective interpretations of situations are the norm, these interpretations become problematic when they repeatedly contribute to maladaptive behaviors, self-critical judgments, and extreme emotion. Take, for example, the patient who notices a young man staring at her in a department store. How she reacts to this situation is entirely dependent on how she interprets this man's attention. If, for example, she thinks, "He must think I look attractive; this is my most flattering outfit after all," she may then smile at the man and feel happy for a short time that afternoon. Conversely, if the patient thinks to herself, "He must think I look so fat in these jeans," she is likely to feel embarrassed and may ruminate about her appearance for the afternoon. Her original thought may fuel additional negative automatic thoughts, such as "I need to lose weight to be attractive," "If I don't lose weight I'll be alone forever," "I must start dieting immediately," and "I will cut out all carbohydrates and fats this week." The patient's original thought also determines her subsequent behavior, which feeds back into the situation and can elicit reinforcement of her original interpretation of the event. For example, if this patient scowls at the man in response to his attention, she may then receive an objectively negative response from him that seemingly confirms her original negative belief that men find her unattractive. Identifying these problematic interpretations (or negative automatic thoughts) is an important component of long-term change.

A–B–C–D Technique

The A-B-C-D technique—identifying the Activating event, Beliefs, Consequences, and Distortions—is a useful way for patients to become more aware of their problematic automatic thoughts that occur between sessions, which will later be challenged with the therapist's assistance. The A-B-C-D technique should be introduced and practiced in **session 8.** Patients often find it useful to watch for strong negative emotions or symptomatic behaviors (*consequences* such as anxiety or bingeing) as a sign that negative automatic thoughts (*beliefs*) just arose. Patients can then work backward to identify the *activating event* that occurred just prior to this reaction as well as any additional *beliefs* related to that situation. Next, patients should review the handout Categories of Distorted Automatic Thoughts: A Guide for Patients (Form 4.8), noticing any biases that may be present in their evaluation of the situation. Each of these A-B-C-D elements can be recorded on the A-B-C-D Technique worksheet (Form 4.9). Identifying cognitive distortions is particularly useful for patients because it allows them some distance from their interpretation and enables them to recognize destructive patterns in their thinking. Patients may find themselves evaluating negative automatic thoughts simply by **labeling the distortion:** "There I go again, *personalizing* her reaction during the meeting." Other examples are shown in Form 4.10.

Thoughts about Food, Dieting, and Control

After identifying and recording their negative automatic thoughts and associated cognitive distortions for a full week, patients may easily recognize the patterns in their thinking. The negative automatic thoughts experienced by patients with BN tend to fall into three categories: (1) beliefs about food, dieting, and control; (2) beliefs about one's own appearance; and (3) beliefs about oneself in relation to others.

A patient's thoughts about food, dieting, and control typically reflect an overgeneralized view that control over food is paramount, certain foods are bad and should be avoided, and (paradoxically) food is a useful emotional coping tool. Examples of such thoughts include: "Controlling my food intake proves I am a good, strong person"; "Potato chips are bad"; "I need to make up for that heavy lunch by skipping dinner"; "I've had a bad day, I deserve a slice of cake"; "I've already blown it, I might as well binge"; "Urges last forever"; and "Bingeing is the only comfort when I'm lonely."

Thoughts about Appearance

Patients also have strong, shameful, and often biased thoughts about appearance, such as: "Being thin is the most important thing"; "I can only be attractive if I'm thin"; "I am inadequate and flawed"; "My stomach should be completely flat"; "I'm a fat pig"; and "I feel so bloated after that binge, I must have gained 5 pounds." Thoughts about appearance, in particular, reflect a dichotomized view of oneself and of the world.

Thoughts about Self in Relation to Others

In addition, patients with BN often unfairly compare themselves with others, engaging in a near-constant internal dialogue about their own weaknesses while glorifying others' attributes. These thoughts about self in relation to others may include: "I'm not any good at this job"; "I must do everything perfectly or else I'm a failure"; "I'll be abandoned if I don't please others"; and "I should be thinner than every other woman in the room."

Once the patient is adept at recognizing her negative automatic thoughts, she is ready to begin cognitive restructuring in session. Cognitive restructuring involves evaluating the automatic thought in a systematic way in order to generate a "rational response," which is a modified interpretation that is less destructive, is less biased, and better reflects the available evidence. With time and practice, cognitive restructuring allows the patient to internalize new thought patterns and more balanced, adaptive beliefs. This technique also is used to help the patient develop more flexible, realistic standards for her body shape, beliefs about certain foods, and interpretations about interactions with others.

Evaluating Automatic Thoughts and Assumptions

Over the course of the next several treatment sessions (**sessions 9–11**), the patient will learn to effectively evaluate, test, and modify her negative automatic thoughts to further disrupt the cycle of her eating disorder. The goal of cognitive restructuring is not positive thinking, nor is it intended to convince the patient that her thoughts are inaccurate and illogical. Rather, the goal is to carefully evaluate the support for and against the negative automatic thoughts, to identify other possible interpretations of the situation, to arrive at a more balanced thought (when warranted), and to reduce the patient's repetitive distorted views of herself and others. There are multiple effective ways to test negative automatic thoughts, and the therapist can demonstrate each of these in session with the patient. Several cognitive restructuring techniques are described next.

Advantages/Disadvantages

Because all situations, interactions, and beliefs about oneself are at least somewhat ambiguous and subjective, it is useful to recognize that we could choose to think differently. Patients are often unaware that they consistently interpret certain situations in a way that contributes to their eating disorder, results in bad feelings, and/or disrupts their interpersonal relationships. To begin the process of thinking differently, patients need to be aware of why it is to their benefit to do so. In short, are there any disadvantages to believing these recurring negative thoughts? Are there any clear advantages? Where does this type of thinking get me? For example, does this type of thinking contribute to feeling worse about myself, to withdrawing from others, and to binge-ing and purging? Does it help me function better or does it contribute to more problems? Would it be to my benefit to believe this thought or, instead, some alternative thought? Which way of thinking makes me feel better in the end?

Selective Attention

Patients often become selectively attuned to information consistent with their negative beliefs about themselves, others, and food. This selective attention to certain details then results in find-ing reinforcement for their negative automatic thoughts. They may *discount positive* information while only paying attention to negative information, resulting in a skewed interpretation of a situation. For example, they may remember only those days last week when they felt unattractive and bloated, not those moments when they were relaxed and felt attractive. Thus, to reframe a negative automatic thought, patients find it useful to be aware of their own biases in attention. They may prompt themselves by asking, "Are there any other facts (present or historical) that I am ignoring or discounting?" "Were there any times that this situation ended differently?"

Automatic Thought Records

As patients become more practiced at stepping back from their automatic thoughts, and become more aware of the emotional and behavioral consequences of their thinking, they are ready to begin formally challenging these thoughts. The most traditional method of cognitive restructur-ing utilizes the seven-column Automatic Thought Record (Form 4.11), on which patients list the concrete, factual evidence that supports and does not support their interpretation of the situation. The goal of these thought records lies in the final column, where patients rewrite their original thoughts in a more balanced, less biased way that reflects the evidence collected on the form. Automatic thought records are simply a structured method of analyzing, challenging, and rewriting negative thoughts related to specific situations. This process can be completed in the moment or, as is often the case with beginners, retrospectively. With practice, this process will become internalized, and patients will learn to challenge their thinking quite readily in the moment.

To complete the automatic thought record, patients begin with the A-B-C-D technique, which they practiced previously. Patients then complete the next two columns, identifying as many pieces of evidence as possible. Patients are often quite skilled at identifying evidence in support of their thoughts but may need prompting to identify nonsupporting evidence. To facilitate this, patients should be asked to consider how this situation has ended in the past, whether others have reacted differently to similar situations, whether there are any alternative ways of viewing this situation, and whether there are any facts (however small) that are not consistent with the automatic thought. In collecting evidence, patients need to watch for their subjective interpretations of the situation and instead only record objective facts. The recorded thought "Even though I had a strong urge, I have not purged on a few occasions" is a factual statement that calls upon the patient's past experiences in similar situations and thus is a good example of evidence against thought. Alternatively, the recorded thought "The urge feels like it will never go away on its own" is not objective evidence but simply another negative automatic thought.

To write the rational balanced response, patients should think about rewriting their negative automatic thoughts as a less definitive, less extreme statement that better reflects the evidence collected. Patients will also want to consider how the situation could end differently if they chose to think differently. A sample completed form pertaining to the case example is included in Chapter 5 (see Figure 5.6).

Rating Belief

When patients first begin using automatic thought records, they often comment that, although they came up with a rational balanced response, they just do not believe this new thought. They tend to think of their original thought and the new response in all-or-nothing terms, contending that they believe one and not the other. Instead of discounting the rational response altogether, patients can be encouraged to rate the degree to which they believe it. This represents a more balanced view of the alternative interpretation rather than the all-or-nothing bias. The therapist also can point out to patients that no matter how small their belief in the rational response, it still represents some movement away from the original automatic thought. Prior to challenging the negative automatic thought, patients likely believed it completely. If there is even a minor belief in the rational response, this indicates that another perspective is viable. With this method, patients also can monitor changes in their beliefs over time and will likely find that the rational responses become more convincing with repetition.

Using a Different Lens

When patients have difficulty identifying alternative evidence for their automatic thoughts, or when they prefer a shorthand way to challenge thoughts in the moment, using "a different lens" is a helpful technique. With this exercise, patients are asked to step outside of their personal experience, and thus their typical interpretation of a situation, and to instead view the situation from a different perspective. This frees patients from their usual biases and long-standing beliefs, allowing room for more objective observation of the circumstances. Patients should ask themselves: "How would a friend see this?" "What advice would I give a friend facing this situation?" "Have other people reacted differently to a similar situation?" "If this was happening to someone else, would I judge them the same way?" "If I was watching this in a movie rather than in my own life, how would I describe what I'm observing?" The answers to these questions help patients arrive more quickly at a rational balanced response.

Behavioral Experiments

A final strategy for challenging negative automatic thoughts is to test them out. This strategy is particularly useful when the patient is unable to identify evidence against her thoughts because she has consistently avoided a situation or behavior. For example, a patient may believe that eating a normal meal with friends will be incredibly uncomfortable, will result in judgment, and will lead to later overeating. The patient may have consistently avoided social eating and thus have little or no evidence against her original thoughts. The patient and therapist can then devise an experiment together in which the patient will not act on her automatic thought but instead act against it (e.g., have dinner with friends rather than avoid it), noting whether the situation turns out as predicted. The result is a collection of new, previously unavailable evidence for cognitive restructuring that can be used in future automatic thought records. The therapist may need to help the patient to not dichotomize the outcome of her experiment, but to instead see the outcome along a continuum with successes, disappointments, and possible areas for improvement.

Food Rules

Aside from negative automatic thoughts, another specific target of cognitive restructuring is the patient's "food rules," those rigid, idiosyncratic, and often dichotomized ideas about specific foods and food intake. These include imperative and moralistic statements, such as "shoulds" about eating and appearance. A patient with BN may believe, for example, that she should not consume any foods after 8 P.M., should always eat less than those around her, should never eat between meals, should completely avoid cakes and other fattening foods, should never eat peanut butter, and should not consume liquid calories. The rigidity of these food rules reflects the patient's excessive pursuit of thinness and, when these rules are broken even slightly, often sets the patient up to binge. In short, these food rules clearly perpetuate dichotomized, disordered eating behaviors and thinking patterns. The therapist and patient should complete the Food Rules Worksheet (Form 4.12) in **session 10,** together listing the patient's specific avoided foods and food rules, using past food records and binge occasions as reminders. Remember, food rules include all foods the patient restricts, avoids, or considers "bad." Each of the food rules should then be ranked relative to one another, with the patient indicating the degree to which she avoids and fears each one.

Prior to disrupting the food rules, it is useful to discuss with the patient **the advantages and disadvantages** of holding such rigid beliefs about food. The therapist can refer the patient to the cognitive-behavioral model of eating disorders (Figure 2.1). The therapist may also ask the patient whether these food rules have effectively served their purpose—does she now feel in control of her eating, has she met her food intake goals, and do they prevent overeating? Conversely, is the patient even more obsessed with thoughts of food now that she holds these food rules, and/or do these rules make her feel abnormal and act differently from others?

The goal of this stage of treatment, which usually takes place during **sessions 11–13,** is the **incremental removal of food rules** and the **reincorporation of restricted foods** into the diet. Food rules interventions proceed in much the same way as exposure and response prevention for obsessive-compulsive disorder (see Leahy, Holland, & McGinn, 2012). The exposure hierarchy, which is a ranked list of food rules, has already been created with the patients. Most are sufficiently motivated to remove or relax their food rules, although they typically fear that doing so will feel too overwhelming, that they will resume bingeing, or that doing so will result in weight gain. Thus, each step of the food rules hierarchy is approached as an **experiment in relaxing food rules,** allowing patients to gradually reincorporate foods without subsequent safety behaviors and to simultaneously test their fears of losing control. When reincorporating restricted foods and when breaking food rules, patients should be instructed to **create a specific plan** in advance to allow exposure while reducing the chances of a subsequent binge–purge. The plan should detail what food rule will be broken, at what time, and with what quantity of food. Patients also may find it useful to **plan distracting or relaxing activities** for later in the day to further prevent the likelihood of bingeing. Last, patients must be sure to resume normal eating for the remainder of the day and the following day to offset any temptation to restrict. It is generally advisable for patients to break one food rule daily on their own between sessions, gradually working up the hierarchy to the most avoided foods and situations. Initial or particularly difficult exposure exercises can occur in therapy sessions, if desired. Patients can **log their exposures** on their daily food records, noting the rule, their anxiety levels, and the outcome. As they develop greater comfort with eating formerly restricted foods, they will no longer need to intentionally add them to their diet on a daily basis, but they should ensure that their eating remains flexible and comfortable (see Relapse Prevention Interventions later in this chapter for more discussion).

As one step to reincorporate restricted foods, a common plan is for a patient to add a portion-controlled package of a forbidden food to her usual lunch. For example, the patient may plan in advance to have a small bag of potato chips in addition to her usual lunch of a soup and salad. Together with the therapist, the patient will make the decision to buy the small bag of potato chips from the deli so that her portion is limited. This will prevent her from losing control and overeating potato chips. After eating her usual lunch and the potato chips, the patient will plan to run an errand in order to distract herself and stay busy for the remainder of her lunch break. The patient will also prepare herself in advance to challenge any thoughts that she has "blown it," that she should now binge, or that she must purge to prevent weight gain. If the patient feels very anxious or upset after consuming the potato chips, she can do several minutes of deep breathing to calm herself. She can also remind herself that these negative feelings will pass within an hour, as she has learned from riding out other urges to purge after a binge. She will also be prepared to have her usual afternoon snack, an apple, in the office and to challenge any temptation to restrict later in the day to compensate for consuming the forbidden food. After carrying out this planned experiment with potato chips, the patient will then record the food intake, her anxiety levels, and any additional comments on her daily food record.

Perfectionism

Perfectionism is a common trait among patients with eating disorders including BN (Fairburn et al., 2003). It has also been linked to a variety of other mental health problems, including depression, social anxiety, and generalized anxiety disorder. Perfectionism is often defined as holding high personal standards, only seeing value in tasks completed perfectly, hiding one's flaws from others, and an inability to tolerate mistakes. Perfectionistic standards can be held for oneself, for others, or both. Patients with an eating disorder are uniquely likely to report elevated concern over making mistakes (Bulik et al., 2003). Individuals with BN often believe that they will be accepted and loved by others only if they maintain perfection in physical appearance, social interactions, school/job performance, and hobbies. Perfectionistic patients often approach hobbies and social interactions to attain success rather than for enjoyment.

The process of adapting perfectionistic standards parallels other cognitive and behavioral interventions: Note the costs of holding these standards, experiment with alternative behaviors, challenge rigid beliefs, and adopt more balanced thought patterns. These interventions are introduced and practiced in **sessions 13–16,** which encompasses both the second and third phases of treatment. Perfectionism is addressed as it relates to food intake, personal standards, and body image.

The patient's idiosyncratic perfectionistic standards, and the costs of maintaining these standards, should first be identified. A patient may note, for example, that perfectionism prevents her from ever feeling satisfied with her performance. The patient may believe that she can always do better, thus becoming overworked. In addition, although the patient may often recognize the ways in which perfectionism contributes to anxiety and eating disorder symptoms, she may also perceive perfectionism as advantageous because it prevents mistakes, maintains control, and ensures consistent approval from others. It is often useful for the therapist to highlight that full recovery from an eating disorder is difficult if the patient changes only her behaviors and fails to change her perfectionistic beliefs.

As with other cognitive restructuring interventions, patients should begin identifying specific perfectionistic thoughts and the associated **cognitive distortions.** In particular, patients should watch for discounting positives, negative filter, and "shoulds." A common (albeit broad) perfectionistic thought that arises among patients with BN is, "If I make a mistake in any aspect of my life, others will no longer respect and like me." Perfectionistic thoughts can then be challenged and revised using the same **cognitive restructuring** techniques described in the previous section.

Another particularly useful intervention is the "double-standard technique," in which patients are asked to consider whether they hold others to the same rigid, high standards as they hold themselves. Patients are asked to consider, for example, whether they expect absolute perfection from others, whether they forgive others for making mistakes, and whether a single mistake changes their impression of another person. In the areas in which they are more lenient with others, patients can begin to intentionally revise their standards to do away with this double standard. Specifically, patients will work to adopt more flexible, less strict standards for themselves. Excessively high standards related to work, relationships, and cleanliness are just as important to address in this treatment as are standards related to food intake, bingeing, and appearance.

In adopting less perfectionistic standards, patients also can utilize a semantic technique. For this exercise, patients are instructed to record any **"should" statements** that arise between sessions (e.g., "I should get an A on my upcoming exam"), and to then rewrite each "should" in the alternative form of "I prefer to . . . " Patients often immediately notice the more flexible nature of preference statements and, with practice, will begin to accept these less rigid preferences. Specifically, many patients can replace their perfectionism with a standard of "good enough." The therapist can help patients examine the costs and benefits of accepting "good enough," practice the double-standard technique ("Is it okay for others to be good enough?"), and evaluate how aiming for good enough can help them cope better with inevitable mistakes and setbacks. One concept that has been helpful for some patients is the idea of "successful imperfectionism," which suggests that one can make progress without being perfect and can attain success through small increments of imperfect performance (Leahy, 2005). This empowers patients to be able to function better with imperfection in an imperfect world.

In order for patients to adapt their perfectionistic belief system, they also will need to learn to give themselves credit for less-than-perfect outcomes. Rather than holding a dichotomized view of success (all perfect or a complete failure), patients can develop a more compassionate and balanced stance with themselves. **Zero-point comparisons** is a particularly helpful technique to reduce the dichotomized viewpoint. Through this technique, patients are reminded that their perfectionistic thinking patterns involve upward comparisons. In short, perfectionistic patients compare themselves to 100%. Instead of noticing what went right, patients are critical of and hyperfocused on the negative aspects of their performance. To address this problematic comparative style, patients are asked to instead use zero-point comparisons to evaluate their performance or to notice how far away from 0% they actually were. This involves defining complete failure in a particular arena. Complete failure is extreme. For example, in giving a speech, 0% would include shaking uncontrollably throughout the speech (not just the first 5 minutes), forgetting *all* of the prepared talk, being booed, and the entire audience leaving the room. After defining the zero point, patients should then note all of the ways in which they surpassed zero and (fairly) give a quantitative rating of their performance (see Form 4.13). In this way, patients will learn to compliment themselves for successes and to notice positive outcomes, even if there were minor flaws or mistakes. A wide variety of cognitive therapy techniques can be found in Leahy's (2003) *Cognitive Therapy Techniques: A Practitioner's Guide.*

Finally, patients can be instructed to **experiment with alternative behaviors,** specifically by making intentional mistakes. Experimentation allows patients to habituate to the discomfort arising from imperfection and to test whether actual outcomes are in line with their fears and beliefs. These experiments can be conducted in a graded manner, similar to the exposure hierarchy for food rules. Seven-column automatic thought records can be completed afterward to record patients' anticipatory fears, actual outcomes (supportive and nonsupportive evidence), and a revised statement about imperfect performances.

Redefining "Healthy"

A cognitive tool to reinforce positive changes and to encourage further behavioral change is to have the patient redefine "healthy." This intervention is useful during **session 14.** During the early stages of an eating disorder, often the patient adapts her diet to include more low-fat foods, fewer empty calories, and more nutritious options. Although these initial changes reflect good health, over time they become more extreme and more rigid. The patient often recognizes that what started as healthy has now become "too healthy," thereby ironically making her unhealthy. At the same time, she may have engaged in these restrictive practices for so long that she has forgotten what constitutes a moderate, healthy diet and lifestyle. Her health applies not only to food intake but also to body weight, physical exercise, body image, interests and hobbies, ability to socialize, level of functioning, and mood. The patient and therapist can together brainstorm a new definition of healthy, both as it specifically applies to the patient and as it would apply to others. Sample responses are shown in Table 4.1. This exercise not only highlights any lingering

TABLE 4.1. Sample Responses to Redefine "Healthy"

1. Body weight at which a person eats an overall healthy diet and exercises moderately
2. Eats three meals and two snacks on most days
3. Feels fairly comfortable with body shape most of the time
4. Can tolerate skipping a day at the gym
5. Enjoys eating out with friends
6. Eats when hungry
7. Wears a bathing suit at the beach or pool
8. Able to indulge like others at the holidays
9. Able to enjoy favorite foods with little or no guilt
10. Does not have restricted foods or unusual food rules
11. Rarely, if ever, binges
12. Has interests and activities unrelated to food/exercise
13. Can cope with stressful situations without bingeing
14. Has supportive friendships
15. Is able to concentrate at work

problems for the patient but also serves as a starting point for discussing long-term maintenance, relapse prevention, and broader life goals. After all, the goal of treatment is not simply to reduce eating disorder symptoms but also to restore physical health and to return the patient to a higher level of functioning and life satisfaction.

BODY IMAGE INTERVENTIONS

Distress over and dissatisfaction with one's body are characteristic of all the eating disorders. The patient with BN, as with any eating disorder, typically judges herself largely by her appearance, expects bodily perfection, may be dissatisfied with her shape, and goes to great lengths to alter or maintain her physical appearance. She may report satisfaction with her appearance and shape but only because she is at a low body weight. She remains terrified of weight gain. The patient's poor body image plays a key role in all facets of her eating disorder, including her cognitions, emotions, dietary restriction, and bingeing and purging behaviors. The patient's perfectionistic expectations and poor body image are especially intertwined. Therefore, as the patient is modifying her rigid perfectionistic expectations in treatment, body image interventions are simultaneously warranted.

The third phase of treatment includes techniques to improve body image, which can be introduced during **session 14.** Body image interventions include (1) addressing the maladaptive thinking patterns that contribute to poor body image; (2) decreasing body-checking and avoidance behaviors; (3) normalizing the presence of physical flaws; (4) lessening the importance of shape/weight as a measure of self-worth; and (5) improving the patient's satisfaction with her body. All of the cognitive restructuring and perfectionism interventions already discussed (e.g., labeling the distortion, zero-point comparisons, and using a different lens) can be used to challenge body image-related cognitions. In addition, several new interventions are useful, discussed next.

The Subjective Nature of Body Image

It is important for the therapist and patient to start body image interventions (**session 14**) by discussing the subjective nature of body image, particularly how perceptions of one's body (or of others' bodies) are open to biases and distortions. Typically, the patient is quick to recognize that body image is not an objective measure of appearance but is instead highly variable and subjective depending on her mood and environment. If, for example, a patient has observed an attractive friend engaged in self-criticism, then she can understand the subjective nature of body image. Furthermore, body image is often biased in that a patient can "feel fat" (emotional reasoning), although her body weight may be low/normal and others perceive her as thin. A patient may also "feel fat" for several hours after a heavy meal or after breaking a food rule, although her body weight cannot actually change this rapidly. Negative thoughts about one's body are reinforced when the patient compares herself against unrealistic standards for her body shape, either by adopting media portrayals of thinness or through self-other comparisons. Throughout the week following session 14, it is useful to have the patient notice (and, if desired, keep a written list of) those events, thoughts, and emotions that trigger poor body image. These triggers will then be reviewed in session 15 and challenged with cognitive restructuring exercises.

Body-Checking and Avoidance Behaviors

Repetitive body-checking behaviors (e.g., pinching fat, critiquing oneself in the mirror) are clear contributors to poor body image because they keep patients hyperfocused on their body shape. In addition, patients typically check certain areas of their body with a critical eye while ignoring others, thus engaging in a cycle of selective attention and confirmation of their negative beliefs. Similarly, patients may intentionally avoid exposing certain body parts (e.g., wearing skirts/shorts, sexual interactions) out of embarrassment or fear of judgment. This avoidance serves as mental confirmation for the patients that they do, in fact, have something to hide, and it prevents receiving positive feedback that could discount their negative beliefs. Thus, identifying (and later adapting) patients' body-checking and avoidance behaviors is a crucial step in improving body image. The **Body Image Checklist** (Appendix B.4; Cooper, Fairburn, & Hawker, 2003) is an excellent self-report tool to assess the presence and extent of body dissatisfaction and checking and avoidance behaviors, and this can be administered during or just prior to **session 14.** Patients often better recognize their problematic thoughts and behaviors after completion of this assessment, and the responses are a useful starting point for behavioral change.

After completing the Body Image Checklist, the patient should be asked to choose one checking behavior to discontinue (or decrease, if necessary) over the coming week. For example, the patient may elect to stop pinching her waist or to limit looking in the mirror to twice daily. Definitions for moderate, reasonable levels of checking may need to be defined in advance. Over the course of the next several treatment sessions, the patient will be asked to progressively **discontinue all excessive body-checking behaviors** and to **begin entering avoided situations.** This exercise will, in the long run, enable the patient to devote less attention to body weight/shape, to reduce the mental focus on thinness, and to possibly obtain more positive feedback. This feedback can then be used as additional evidence for cognitive restructuring. As the patient successfully modifies her body-checking and avoidance behaviors, her preoccupation with and dissatisfaction with her shape and weight are also likely to decrease significantly. How the patient will change these behaviors and any anticipated difficulties while doing so should be problem solved proactively with the therapist in session.

Cognitive Restructuring of Body Image

Session 15, as with all sessions, should begin with a review of the patient's homework from the previous week. In particular, reviewing the patient's body image triggers will set the stage for cognitive change exercises in the current session. After noting in the last session that body image is a subjective and highly variable quality, the patient should be better able to disengage from her negative thoughts about her body, which will then allow her to begin questioning the validity of these thoughts. By noting her body image triggers over the past week, the patient will have a clearer idea of when and where these destructive thoughts arise. **Session 15** can, therefore, be devoted, in part, to cognitive restructuring, which is the process of evaluating and adapting these negative thoughts. The seven-column technique for cognitive restructuring, as described earlier, involves identifying unrealistic and distorted shape-related thoughts, considering evidence for and against these thoughts, revising these thoughts to better reflect the gathered evidence, and ultimately adopting a more compassionate and realistic view of her body (see Form 4.11). Cognitive restructuring should be practiced in session and assigned as ongoing homework between treatment sessions.

Unrealistic Standards

Also in **session 15,** the therapist and patient will explicitly discuss the ways in which the patient places too much emphasis on her physical appearance and holds herself to unrealistic body standards. The patient may acknowledge that, despite making multiple changes thus far in treatment, she still thinks about her body shape throughout the day and is unable to concentrate on much else. In addition, she may note that she values her appearance above all other qualities, continues to believe that a "perfect" body is attainable, or believes that she would be permanently distressed were she to require a larger clothing size. The explicit goal at this stage is for the patient to allow that physical imperfections are inevitable, normal, and tolerable, and that other aspects of herself are at least equally (if not more) important than her appearance. One way to begin shifting her priorities is to have the patient outline all the perceived **advantages and disadvantages of aspiring for a "perfect" body** versus accepting that physical flaws are normal (see Form 4.14). The patient's eating disorder has served as a way to maintain (perceived) control over her appearance and body, and thus "letting go" of these standards and behaviors can be very scary. The patient believes that letting her guard down even a little will result in rapid and uncontrolled weight gain. Thus, maintaining control is a commonly noted advantage of continuing to strive for perfection. Because the patient commonly expects "more anxiety" and fears "letting myself go" if she reduces her standards, avoidance of these emotions can also be perceived as advantages of continued striving. Significant disadvantages of aspiring for the perfect body may include the obsessions, time, dissatisfaction, extreme dieting, and shame, which are all associated with having an eating disorder. Commonly cited advantages of forgoing a perfect body include: more time to focus on other interests; able to concentrate at work again; feel less shallow; won't feel controlled by the eating disorder any longer; might be able to feel good about oneself; and could accept compliments from others. Additional cognitive restructuring may be useful here to adapt the patient's beliefs about the feasibility of having a perfect body and about whether she can be happy despite her imperfections. Most patients recognize that others have imperfections but are happy and attractive nonetheless. Again, applying the concept of "successful imperfection" can help the patient make progress toward realistic goals.

Broadening Self–Worth

After devoting approximately half of **session 15** to normalizing and increasing the patient's motivation to accept physical flaws, the remainder of the session can be devoted to helping the patient develop other ways to define her self-worth. The goal is for the patient to simultaneously allow for imperfection while adopting non-appearance-related reasons to feel good about herself. The following intervention will demonstrate how limited the patient's life has become as a result of the eating disorder, and helps encourage the patient to either begin or to continue working toward defining herself in a broader, healthier way. With the therapist's assistance, the patient can complete the **pie chart exercise** (see Form 4.15) on which she visually describes those qualities she deems most important to her self-image. The top portion of this form requires the patient to define those characteristics, roles, and activities that were most important to her at the start of treatment, drawing different size wedges to depict the perceived importance of each. It is not unusual for a patient to report that at least 90% of her self-image was determined by her appearance, while the remaining 10% was equally divided among other important aspects of her life. The bottom portion of the form allows the patient to describe a more balanced view of herself that she can now work toward. The patient should be encouraged to include any personal characteristics, roles, or activities that are important to her or give her satisfaction, for example, intimate relationships; being a good friend; being honest; physical exercise, such as swimming; financial independence; appearance; creative outlets; and career success. The pie chart exercise highlights which factors, beyond appearance, are valued by the patient. Having fixed, even proportions of the eight areas underscores the need to work toward a healthy balance in one's life.

Following completion of the pie chart exercise, a useful homework assignment is for the patient to carry out one activity daily that advances a non-appearance-related area from the pie chart. For example, a patient may decide to improve "creativity," and thus may agree to knit or draw each evening after work. Alternatively, a patient may opt to call an old friend to refocus on her relationships rather than spend those 20 minutes scrutinizing her appearance in the mirror.

Reviewing History

As the patient begins to change her behaviors to reflect a more balanced life, it is important to continue cognitive interventions to loosen her associations between appearance and happiness. Although cognitive restructuring should be utilized steadily beginning in session 9, an additional focused intervention can be introduced during **session 16.** The goal of the following exercise is to raise the patient's awareness that her eating disorder has not brought her control or happiness, that thinness is neither a prerequisite nor a guarantee for happiness, and that her beliefs about shape and weight are often faulty. One way to address these associations and to challenge her related beliefs is to "review history," that is, to review how she felt about herself at various points (specifically at different body weights) in her past. Useful questions to review the patient's past include:

"Was there ever a time when you felt good about your appearance? Why did you feel comfortable? What was your weight at that time? What were your eating habits at that time?"

"When were you at your lowest adult body weight? Did you like yourself then? Were you perfectly happy with your appearance? Did you feel healthy at that weight? Did others think you looked your best?"

"What sacrifices, if any, did you make to be at your lowest body weight? Did this body weight require extreme dieting or compensatory behaviors? Did you feel any shame or embarrassment about how you achieved this low weight?"

"What was your highest adult body weight? When was that? How did you feel about yourself then? Were you objectively overweight or healthy? What did others say?"

"Was there ever a time when you thought relatively little about food? When you obsessed less about your body? When? Why?"

Through this exercise, patients typically discover that they have been continuously dissatisfied with their bodies despite higher and lower past weights. Often patients will describe feeling just as or more dissatisfied when at their lowest body weight as they were at higher weights. Some patients will describe feeling more critical the lower their body weight went. Similarly, some patients realize that they were happiest before their eating disorder began, when they were at a healthy body weight (possibly even slightly overweight), and when they spent relatively little time thinking about their food intake. Some patients remember feeling "flabby" or "disgusting" while at a body weight that they would now consider their ideal. Of course, some patients will have had a history of being overweight and fear returning to that point or, at the other extreme, felt attractive and accomplished at a very low body weight. No matter the history, it is important to review patients' body image at various weights along the continuum and to challenge their belief that lower weights always bring satisfaction. In the end, many patients see that they were never satisfied, no matter how low their body weight was, and that the eating disorder always left them striving for something more. Responses to the prior questions can become evidence for seven-column cognitive restructuring exercises in which the patients challenge their positive or negative beliefs about weight and body image. As homework between sessions 16 and 17, patients should complete several Automatic Thought Records (see Form 4.11) to challenge such beliefs. One particularly important thought to challenge is, "If I get/stay thin, I will be happy." A history of excessive focus on thinness is often associated with anxiety and self-criticism rather than contentment, and this suggests that the relentless pursuit of body image is a hopeless endeavor.

Stopping Unfair Comparisons

Unfair comparisons are a specific type of cognitive distortion that perpetuate negative body image and thus warrant special attention in **session 16.** Patients typically engage in repetitive, unfair comparisons between themselves and others, which reinforce existing negative thoughts about themselves. In almost every instance of self–other comparisons, patients identify a favorable characteristic in another person and then criticize themselves for being less desirable in that area. Patients tend to focus on those characteristics about which they themselves are self-conscious (e.g., their stomach), and then notice others whom they deem more attractive in that area (e.g., selective attention for flat abs). The problem with these comparisons is that they not only make the patient feel worse about herself, but they also are biased and unfair. Patients also tend to draw sweeping conclusions (overgeneralizing) based on these comparisons, such as about the person's happiness, success, or desirability relative to their own. For example, patients may believe that others are always happy and successful, based on their weight, without recognizing that many of these "admired" people also have life problems. It is important to discuss with patients the characteristics in others that they choose to ignore and all the "average" individuals with whom they do not compare themselves. Are these "average people" always miserable? Patients' comparisons are self-destructive specifically because they are so unfair—that is, patients do not factor in their own positive characteristics and others' shortcomings (visible or not) when they make these self–other comparisons. The seven-column cognitive restructuring exercise should be continued as homework following this session, this time challenging these unfair self–other comparisons as well as other negative body image thoughts.

Positive Data Log

As the patient approaches the end of treatment, a final body image intervention can be introduced to directly improve her body image. Feeling better about her appearance and her body will be protective against future relapse. Thus, in **session 17,** the therapist and patient should together begin a positive data log, an ongoing list of evidence in support of positive body image. This list should include anything that supports the positive belief, "My body is beautiful." The patient may log everything that supports this statement, including situations, emotions, compliments received, objective facts, and her own observations. Unlike evidence gathering for the automatic thought records, the patient is not limited to listing concrete, objective facts. The therapist may need to help the patient generate items at first, although the patient will become more adept with daily practice. The positive data log should be kept daily, and duplicate items can be recorded as often as they occur. Commonly listed positive data include, but are not limited to, "Others complimented me on how I looked in this dress today"; "I am at a normal body weight"; "My legs are strong and allow me to climb stairs"; "My boyfriend thinks I'm sexy"; "My hair looks good"; "I have a great smile"; "I like my shoulders"; "A man flirted with me in the grocery store"; "I feel beautiful when I stand up tall."

The patient should complete the log throughout the day, and should periodically review her growing list of positive data. She may wish to set a daily time for reviewing her list, perhaps every evening before bed. This exercise will serve as a reminder of her positive qualities and thus directly bolster self-image. The positive data log also helps improve body image by disrupting the cycle of selective attention, discounting positives, and negative filtering that maintains poor body image. This is accomplished when the patient shifts her focus away from self-criticism and problem areas and onto positive aspects of her appearance. Over time, the patient will likely become more attuned to positive things about herself, her mental focus will shift, and she will spend less time focusing on perceived imperfections.

OPTIONAL SUPPLEMENTARY INTERVENTIONS

As patients near the end of treatment, cognitive and behavioral interventions should continue to be practiced to solidify positive changes. This penultimate stage of treatment also warrants problem solving regarding any lingering eating disorder symptoms and potential difficulties with maintenance. Two common areas in which patients require additional assistance are interpersonal difficulties and emotion regulation. Selected interventions for interpersonal problems and emotion regulation skills are presented in the following sections, and are intended to be used as needed to augment the traditional cognitive-behavioral interventions. **Interpersonal difficulties** that interact with the eating disorder may include, but are not limited to, discomfort with eating in public; lack of trust in intimate relationships; social isolation; lack of social support; difficulties with assertive communication; loss of an important relationship; role transitions; direct or indirect social pressure for thinness; feeling "watched" at meals; and dieting behaviors and diet talk among peers. **Emotion regulation** refers to the ability to identify, to understand, to tolerate, to communicate about, and to effectively channel one's emotions in a healthy, adaptive manner. Patients who have coping skills deficits in this area may find themselves easily overwhelmed by negative or positive emotions, may not understand their emotions and their triggers, may suffer negative consequences as a result of strong emotional responses, may have trouble expressing their emotions in a productive way, and may find it difficult to divert their attention once in distress. Bingeing is thought to be a maladaptive attempt to cope with negative affect among patients with BN (Tanofsky-Kraff & Wilfley, 2010).

Interpersonal difficulties and emotional coping deficits, although not a problem for every patient with BN, may directly or indirectly contribute to bingeing, purging, dietary restriction, or poor body image. These difficulties may also make patients more vulnerable to future relapse. Thus, these potential deficits should be evaluated carefully as part of the cognitive-behavioral model of eating disorders. Interpersonal and emotional difficulties may have predated the eating disorder (e.g., considers negative emotions intolerable), may have developed in conjunction with eating disorder symptoms (e.g., self-consciousness about quantities consumed relative to others), or may have arisen as a coping mechanism during treatment (e.g., avoids coffee shops as a stimulus control measure). Not all patients exhibit interpersonal or emotional difficulties, and thus these should be addressed in a targeted manner and only for those patients for whom it is warranted. In fact, recent research suggests that an expanded cognitive-behavioral protocol that includes interpersonal, self-esteem, perfectionism, and mood intolerance interventions may be more effective than traditional CBT for those patients with these respective difficulties but counterproductive for the remaining patients (Fairburn et al., 2009). Interventions for these areas can be utilized in **sessions 17–18,** depending on patients' current presentation and original case formulation.

Interpersonal Interventions

Interpersonal difficulties are common among patients with eating disorders and, like CBT, IPT has been found to be effective in the treatment of BN (Agras, Walsh, et al., 2000). IPT is a short-term psychological treatment focused on specific interpersonal problem areas that are thought to contribute directly or indirectly to the eating disorder (Tanofsky-Kraff & Wilfley, 2010). In IPT, the interpersonal problems themselves, and not the eating disorder symptoms, are the target of treatment. It is thought that the severity and frequency of bingeing, purging, and restrictive behaviors decrease as patients' interpersonal difficulties are resolved because the patients develop more satisfying relationships, experience less interpersonal distress, have fewer emotional distur-bances, and engage in more activities.

For those therapists using a cognitive-behavioral approach, interpersonal modules can be effectively utilized to augment the traditional CBT protocol. These interpersonal modules can address any social skills deficits and problems in the social network (Fairburn et al., 2009). Inter-personal interventions should be directly related to patients' case conceptualizations and, like-wise, should be tailored to address patients' specific difficulties in relationship functioning. Thus, the same interventions will not be utilized with all patients. The goal of the interpersonal inter-ventions, as with all others for the eating disorder, is to move patients toward healthier, more balanced functioning in all areas of life.

In evaluating which interpersonal difficulties to address at this stage of treatment, the thera-pist should consider the following four problem areas that are typically addressed in IPT: grief, interpersonal role disputes, role transitions, and interpersonal deficits (Fairburn, 1997; Tanofsky-Kraff & Wilfley, 2010). Problems with grief can arise after the death of a loved one or the loss of a significant relationship. Interpersonal role disputes refer to relationship conflict that stems from differing expectations about a relationship or problems communicating one's expectations. Difficulties with role transitions can occur if patients do not adjust to a change in life roles, such as the birth of a child or a career change. Interpersonal deficits refer to extreme social isolation, a pattern of unfulfilling relationships, or an inability to develop or maintain relationships. Inter-personal role disputes are most commonly experienced by patients with BN (present in 64% of patients), followed by role transitions (36%), interpersonal deficits (16%), and grief (12%; Fair-burn, 1997).

Although interpersonal binge triggers will have been addressed in prior CBT treatment ses-sions, only one or two treatment sessions are devoted solely to resolving residual interpersonal problems. Thus, it is advisable to select one interpersonal problem area to work on in sessions 17 and 18. However, the therapist and patient can also expand the number of sessions to help the patient cope with interpersonal problems. In IPT, the therapist and patient also typically work on the one interpersonal problem area most closely related to the eating disorder (Tanofsky-Kraff & Wilfley, 2010). For example, a patient may continue to feel urges to binge following frequent fights with her boyfriend. The next two treatment sessions could then target this interpersonal role dispute. Alternatively, a patient may no longer binge but remains socially isolated. If loneli-ness was a common binge precipitant for this patient at the start of treatment, the therapist may wish to address this interpersonal deficit to reduce the patient's chance of future relapse.

As in IPT, sessions 17 and 18 of the current protocol should be supportive, nondirective, and focused on how the patient can effectively resolve a specific interpersonal difficulty. Further, the therapist should encourage the patient to take the lead in resolving this identified problem area. IPT does not utilize specific techniques as in CBT, but does require a focused and collaborative problem-solving style to guide the patient toward improving her interpersonal situations. In sessions 17 and 18, the therapist may utilize any one or more of the approaches described next to target specific interpersonal difficulties related to the patient's eating disorder. As with CBT, these interpersonal interventions are used to guide the patient toward change, with the understanding that the patient will continue to make further progress on her own once treatment ends.

If interpersonal interventions are to be used in sessions 17 and 18, the therapist may wish to begin with a **discussion of the interpersonal context** in which the patient's eating disorder symptoms were developed and maintained. This will help orient the patient to the need to address interpersonal problems to ensure a full recovery from the eating disorder, and will help the therapist and patient together prioritize the interpersonal difficulty that most needs to be addressed.

After discussing the interpersonal context of the patient's eating disorder and agreeing on one specific interpersonal target for this stage of treatment, the therapist and patient can move on to a focused discussion of how to resolve this identified interpersonal problem. In-session interventions for interpersonal difficulties will likely include a combination of **communication skills training, cognitive restructuring, problem solving,** and **role plays.** For example, the therapist may help the patient cope with social pressure to overeat by using problem-solving skills, positive coping statements, and food-refusal role plays in session. A patient who views her social network as a trigger for restriction and self-critical thinking, for example, may benefit from challenging her unhealthy comparisons with others, especially as they relate to body image, dieting, and exercise.

If the primary identified interpersonal problem is **grief,** the goal of these two modular sessions is to assist the patient with mourning and to then help her move past the grief (Tanofsky-Kraff & Wilfley, 2010). The therapist may start by educating the patient about the grief process, including the expected stages of grief. The patient may also be encouraged to express emotion in session to assist with mourning. The therapist and patient could then challenge any idealization about the deceased loved one or lost relationship. Finally, the therapist and patient may together problem solve how the patient can develop new interests, relationships, and social activities to redevelop a meaningful life.

Interpersonal role disputes are the most common type of interpersonal difficulty experienced by the patient with BN. When the patient's primary identified problem is an **interpersonal role dispute,** the goal is to understand what is maintaining this interpersonal conflict and find a way to resolve it (Fairburn, 1997). The therapist may help the patient improve communication with the other person, either through assertiveness training or role plays. If the interpersonal dispute involves unrealistic expectations of the other person or distorted perceptions about the relationship, the patient may benefit from cognitive restructuring exercises. If the relationship is particularly destructive or interpersonal interventions do not ameliorate the difficulties, it may be necessary for the therapist to help the patient terminate this problematic relationship.

If the patient's primary interpersonal difficulty is in coping with a **role transition,** the therapist will work with the patient to accept this new role (Fairburn, 1997). In sessions 17 and 18, the patient may benefit from challenging any distorted perceptions of this new role. This may include an evaluation of the positive and negative aspects of the new role. Further, the patient should be encouraged by the therapist to develop the necessary skills and social support for effectively managing this new role. This may include in-session role plays, problem solving, and communication skills training. Because the patient with BN tends to hide her emotional and practical difficulties from others, the patient and therapist may need to role-play the experience of asking others in the patient's social network for healthy support around this role transition.

When the patient's primary interpersonal difficulty is an **interpersonal deficit,** the goal of sessions 17 and 18 should be to start improving the quality of the patient's current relationships and to help her develop new relationships. The therapist should begin by examining the reasons for the patient's long-standing difficulty developing or maintaining relationships. When social skills deficits are apparent, the therapist may utilize role plays and communication skills training to help the patient become more adept at forming relationships with others. For the patient who has become socially isolated as a consequence of her eating disorder, the goal is to reintegrate the patient in social activities and to resume social eating. To this end, the therapist may utilize behavioral experiments, role plays, and an exposure hierarchy.

Regardless of the interpersonal focus in sessions 17 and 18, the therapist should remember that the goal is to initiate change and to empower the patient to make continued, independent change in improving her interpersonal functioning in the targeted area, even after this stage of treatment is complete.

Emotion Regulation Interventions

Like the interpersonal interventions, emotion regulation interventions are an optional treatment module and, if needed, should be targeted to the patient's current symptoms and case conceptualization. BN can, in part, be conceptualized as a lack of emotional coping skills. Specifically, the patient with BN may have an impaired ability to regulate her distress associated with negative emotions. Thus, the three primary behaviors associated with BN—bingeing, purging, and dieting—can be thought of as maladaptive attempts to control, distract from, or avoid negative emotion. Body image concerns are just one of many possible triggers for a patient's negative emotions. Emotion regulation interventions may, therefore, help the patient to better tolerate distress, to improve her understanding of the function of emotions, and to better anticipate and therefore respond to emotional triggers. The patient may benefit from simply **reframing the eating disorder** as an ineffective attempt at coping with negative emotions, and this in turn will allow the patient to consider other behavioral responses.

For patients with emotion regulation difficulties, **self-soothing skills** should be introduced and practiced. Self-soothing refers to any action (mental or behavioral) that helps patients calm themselves. The goal is typically to transition from a negative to a neutral mood state or to at least decrease the intensity of the emotion. Self-soothing skills are useful for individuals experiencing any negative emotion, anxiety, stress, tearfulness, or loss of control, and they can be particularly useful for interrupting binges (Safer et al., 2001). Common self-soothing techniques include (1) diaphragmatic breathing; (2) urge surfing; (3) use of positive affirmations; (4) engaging in a distracting activity; (5) "opposite action"; and (6) coping cards. Any combination of these self-soothing skills can be taught in sessions 17 and 18.

Diaphragmatic breathing, a strategy introduced in session 6, was previously described as a behavioral alternative to bingeing. Patients may find it useful to review this skill and to practice it both in and between sessions for use as a more general coping strategy. Ideally, patients will practice the breathing exercises daily to feel adequately prepared for use in difficult, emotional situations. Taking slow, deep breaths while keeping the mind focused will allow both physiological and mental relaxation to occur.

Urge surfing, another binge alternative first introduced in session 5, can be modified and used again at this stage of treatment to help the patient "ride out" negative emotions. Urge surfing is a mindfulness technique and thus is appropriate for learning to better tolerate distressing emotions in addition to cravings. As with all mindfulness techniques, the goal is for the patient to neither block the emotion nor to get rid of it, but to allow it in without struggling against it and to, therefore, incur fewer negative consequences (e.g., without acting on it, without bingeing to numb the emotion, or with less distress or feeling less overwhelmed because of the emotion). Emotions, like urges, also can be triggered easily, often come on seemingly suddenly, build in intensity until they peak, will ultimately pass if left alone, and simply reflect an internal experience, not a mandate to act. When faced with a strong negative emotion, the patient should be instructed to first notice and label her emotion (e.g., "I am feeling angry"), and then to visualize herself riding the emotion through its rise, crest, and fall. While surfing the emotion, the patient remembers that although the emotion is powerful, it only knocks her down if she fights against it. If, instead, the patient allows the emotion to come and go, she can emerge on the other side with minimal damage to herself and others. Thus, this modified form of urge surfing can enable the patient to better tolerate emotional distress.

While experiencing a negative emotion, the patient often exacerbates her distress by becoming self-critical about the way in which she is handling the situation, other people, and her emotions. A patient may say to herself, "Only weak people get so upset about these kinds of things" or "I should have been able to stay completely calm." Such negative self-statements then add additional upset or anxiety onto the original situation, and leave the patient feeling more distressed and vulnerable. Instead, the therapist and patient can practice self-validation, which entails using **positive affirmations** in the face of overwhelming negative emotion. In session, the therapist and patient can together generate a list of potential affirmative statements to be used when in distress, which may include:

"It makes sense that I reacted strongly to this situation."

"If a friend were in this situation, I wouldn't be surprised if she reacted in the same way."

"Feeling angry is not the same as acting on my anger."

"Although I was upset, I was able to contain it and move on from it."

"I used good coping strategies, like deep breathing, to get through that."

"Negative emotions always feel like they will last forever, but they usually subside within a half-hour."

Another useful self-soothing skill is to deliberately **engage in a distracting activity.** It is difficult to remain focused on two things simultaneously, so a new, engaging activity may help the patient forget (or at least lessen) the original distress. Any activity should work because it will both occupy her mind with something else and allow enough time to pass for the emotion to subside (e.g., riding it out). The best activities are those that fully engage the mind, require sustained concentration, and utilize all five senses (e.g., playing with a child vs. watching television). Activities that are incompatible with the original emotion are also effective. Intentionally choosing a behavior that elicits the opposite emotion is referred to as **"opposite action."** Opposite action may include calling a friend when feeling lonely, taking a hot shower or bath when anxious, watching a funny sitcom while sad, or completing a task when feeling ineffective.

Because it is important for the patient to practice self-soothing techniques regularly between sessions (particularly *in vivo* whenever possible), **coping cards** (see Form 4.16) can be generated in advance to ensure that the patient remembers to use her designated self-soothing skills. Coping cards are useful for recurring or anticipated difficult situations that allow the patient to problem solve in advance. To complete a coping card, the patient and therapist first define the anticipated situation and then together generate a list of alternative behavioral, cognitive, and emotional responses to use in the situation. Afterward, the patient agrees to carry the coping card with her to consult when the situation occurs.

Many patients have negative beliefs about their emotions, viewing their anxiety or distress as shameful, out of control, overwhelming, unique to them, lasting forever, and not making any sense (Leahy, 2002). These are their **"emotional schemas"**—that is, their attributions for emotions, explanations, and evaluations. Because binge eating and purging are often triggered by difficulty coping with emotions, patients can be assisted in dealing with these problematic emotional schemas. Patients with negative beliefs about emotion are more likely to use problematic strategies to suppress their emotions, such as bingeing, purging, abusing substances, and self-harm. However, these patients may be assisted in modifying their negative beliefs to learn more adaptive and realistic beliefs and strategies. For example, they may recognize that many other people have the same emotions; their emotions make sense given their negative thoughts about themselves; emotions come and go in intensity; suppressing emotions only makes them feel more intense; there is nothing evil about having a feeling; and once emotions are accepted, tolerated, and observed in a mindful and dispassionate manner, they often subside. Further discussion of emotional schemas and other emotion regulation strategies can be found in *Emotion Regulation in Psychotherapy: A Practitioner's Guide* (Leahy, Tirch, & Napolitano, 2011).

RELAPSE PREVENTION INTERVENTIONS

By this final phase of treatment, the majority of patients either will have achieved complete remission from BN or will have markedly reduced many of their eating disorder symptoms, including dietary restriction, problematic food rituals and rules, bingeing, purging, harmful cognitions, poor body image, and insufficient or maladaptive coping skills. Posttreatment recovery rates are estimated to be 50% with traditional CBT, with another 30% of patients achieving a significant reduction in symptoms (Keel & Mitchell, 1997). The explicit goal of CBT is not simply to treat the eating disorder symptoms in an effective and efficient manner, but also to help patients learn the skills required to maintain these improvements over the long term. Approximately 30% of patients who have improved or recovered through treatment will later relapse (Keel & Mitchell, 1997). Thus, the final stage of treatment, typically comprising **sessions 19 and 20,** is devoted to relapse prevention. Relapse prevention, in this instance, refers to the review and reinforcement of skills learned throughout treatment, planning ahead for setbacks, and a discussion about when further treatment is warranted, all of which should help ensure that patients' eating disorders do not resurface in the future.

Reviewing Treatment Interventions

In order to prevent a relapse to eating disorder behaviors, it is important for the patient to be aware of her past triggers, to learn to prevent and/or manage these triggers on an ongoing basis, and to identify a viable early response strategy should a setback or full relapse occur. To begin, the therapist and patient should review the treatment techniques utilized throughout this course of treatment, especially emphasizing those interventions the patient found most helpful in recovering from her eating disorder. The therapist may want to highlight several interventions that are the cornerstone of CBT: food records, regular eating, and cognitive restructuring. After reviewing the helpful treatment techniques, the patient may wish to create a master list of these cognitive-behavioral interventions to which she can then refer in the future, should it become necessary. In addition, the patient may find it useful to organize her treatment notes and worksheets in a folder so that they are all readily available for future reference.

Listing Past Triggers

The therapist and patient should also together identify and list the patient's idiosyncratic triggers that previously made her vulnerable to bingeing, purging, or dietary restriction. These will include the triggers identified through careful assessment and functional analysis at the start of treatment as well as those that became apparent through daily food monitoring. Because *past triggers tend to later become relapse situations,* it will benefit the patient to be aware of which people, places, emotions, and situations may make her most vulnerable to relapse in the future.

Relapse Roadmap

Once the therapist and patient have determined when and where the patient may be most vulnerable to relapse, and have together discussed the therapeutic techniques available to the patient as a first response, the next step is to create a Relapse Roadmap (Form 4.17). The relapse roadmap is a technique commonly used in CBT for addictions. It is a detailed, personalized plan for how to handle trigger situations, how to get back on track when faced with a setback, which treatment techniques and worksheets will be beneficial to use if symptoms return, and when to return for additional treatment sessions. The relapse roadmap reminds the patient which triggers are potentially most problematic for her, what behavioral and emotional responses would be harmful when faced with those triggers, and what healthier alternatives (e.g., cognitive-behavioral interventions, interpersonal support, coping skills) she has available to her. This worksheet should be completed together with the therapist in the final treatment session. The goal is to bring together all of the tools available to the patient in a solid plan that will be useful after treatment completion. If the patient has a concrete plan for handling setbacks, she may be able to reduce her vulnerability to relapse. The relapse roadmap serves as a reminder that strict dieting, under- or overconsumption of certain foods, untreated depression or anxiety symptoms, poor stress coping skills, and dips in her body image are several possible relapse triggers. In the face of any of these early signs of relapse, which can be thought of as "red flags," the patient should now have a pre-planned coping response to maintain her health and recovery.

Lapse versus Relapse

Prior to termination, the therapist may wish to distinguish a lapse, which is a common occurrence during recovery, from a full-blown relapse to disordered eating behaviors. A **lapse** may include a temporary resumption of dieting, bingeing, or purging but, if addressed quickly, can easily be managed with minimal long-term consequences. A lapse can be thought of as a learning experience, a signal of where the patient remains vulnerable. Lapses are most common during times of high stress and role changes in the patient's life, and they are to be expected. If the patient is aware that a lapse is likely to occur, she may react more positively and cope more efficiently when faced with one. The patient may be able to recover from a lapse on her own by simply following her relapse roadmap. On the other hand, a **relapse** is a prolonged, problematic resumption of the eating disorder. A relapse will include multiple symptoms and consequences that occur over a period of time, with the symptoms gradually increasing in severity just as they did with the disorder's original onset. Because of their severity and intensity, it will be more difficult for the patient to contain a relapse without additional treatment. She will likely feel demoralized and ashamed if faced with a relapse. Thus, it is important that the therapist normalize a lapse, emphasize the importance of correcting lapses early, and stress the need to seek additional treatment if eating disorder symptoms return. The patient should be encouraged to return to treatment for a single or several "booster sessions" whenever necessary so as to maintain her health and progress.

POSSIBLE "ROADBLOCKS" AND TREATMENT RESISTANCE

The majority of patients with BN will, at least once during the course of treatment, find it difficult or anxiety provoking to fully comply with treatment recommendations. Rather than labeling the noncompliance as resistance or lack of motivation, the cognitive-behavioral therapist may find it more useful to conceptualize the patient's noncompliance as a normal, understandable reaction to the prospect of change. In fact, some noncompliance (e.g., continued purging, failure to eat throughout the day, or intense fear of weight gain) simply reflects the symptoms of BN. It is also useful to consider that treatment roadblocks (e.g., continued bingeing or midtreatment setbacks) can be equally frustrating for patient and therapist.

There are several particularly common roadblocks that occur during CBT for BN (see Table 4.2). Roadblocks may stem from patients' fears of gaining weight, of losing control, of setting themselves up for a binge, or of breaking a long-standing food rule. Patients who do not fully accept the cognitive-behavioral model of BN may intentionally attend to some interventions (e.g., those that will disrupt bingeing) while ignoring others (e.g., those that address dietary restriction and food rules). Patients are often reluctant to give up those aspects of their disor-

TABLE 4.2. Common "Roadblocks" in Bulimia Nervosa Treatment

- Frequent tardiness or missed sessions
- Reluctance to keep daily food records
- Failure to eat planned, regular meals and snacks
- Not monitoring and/or challenging automatic thoughts
- General homework noncompliance
- Patient feels hopeless and/or discounts treatment progress
- Continued vomiting or laxative use
- Continued dietary restriction
- Lack of symptom improvement
- Resumption of bingeing and purging after a period of abstinence

der that provide them with the illusion of control and safety. Perfectionism is common among patients with eating disorders, as is a strong desire to obtain approval from others, including their therapist. Patients may, therefore, experience shame when unable to meet their own particularly high expectations. Patients often attempt to hide perceived failures from their therapist (e.g., choose to discontinue food records completely rather than write down a single binge–purge episode), or they take an all-or-nothing approach to treatment compliance (e.g., experience an urge to binge, subsequently feel that treatment is not working, and therefore give up on completing thought records).

Expressing surprise at the first sign of noncompliance is often useful, as is reviewing with patients the importance of homework for solidifying skills development and behavioral change between sessions. Food records and thought records are particularly important for symptom improvement. Patients often resume compliance after a reminder that CBT is deliberately active and collaborative, and that symptom improvement is contingent on homework completion. It is also helpful to review the cognitive-behavioral model of BN and to underscore the necessity of addressing all symptoms. Another quite basic, and often effective, intervention for noncompliance is for the therapist to simultaneously normalize difficulties with homework compliance and to explore patients' reasons for not practicing interventions between sessions. This provides patients with an opportunity to openly vocalize any fears or misunderstandings about the interventions.

Other common therapeutic interventions can be effectively applied to treatment roadblocks and, when addressed soon after they arise, can provide an opportunity to bolster motivation for change, to practice problem solving, and to challenge relevant dysfunctional cognitions. These interventions include the following.

Reviewing Advantages and Disadvantages

When a patient reports feeling "stuck" or unmotivated to practice interventions between sessions, working with her to identify the advantages and disadvantages of doing so can be valuable. In creating this list of pros and cons, the therapist should make sure that the patient includes historical and ongoing consequences of the targeted symptom (e.g., eating in secret creates a feeling of isolation and mistrust from others). The patient will often recognize that she has overestimated the amount of time and energy the assigned homework will require or that the associated discomfort is temporary and is outweighed by the potential gains. A review of the advantages and disadvantages can focus on a particular intervention with which the patient is struggling or on treatment engagement in general.

Behavioral Experiments

Patients with BN, even when highly motivated to recover from their eating disorder, commonly fear letting go of select rigid behaviors and cognitions. They often fear that doing so will cause them to gain weight, to lose control, to become more preoccupied with food, or to binge more frequently. This is particularly common when implementing interventions such as food records, eating on schedule, reincorporating restricted foods, decreasing perfectionistic standards, and body acceptance strategies. When patients are fearful of committing to a certain behavior (e.g., eating three normal-sized meals and two snacks daily), they may be more willing to comply when the intervention is framed as a time-limited experiment (4 weeks is often particularly effective). As an experiment, they are free to resume their old behavior if they find the new one too distressing or ineffective, but only after the agreed-upon trial period.

Challenging Distorted Cognitions

Having the patient identify those cognitive distortions and challenge those negative automatic thoughts that interfere with treatment compliance is an important step. This allows the therapist and patient not only to work through the current roadblock but also to identify broader thinking patterns associated with the eating disorder. Often the patient will recognize that she has negative interpretations about her treatment progress ("I'm not getting better at all") or about the effect of a particular intervention ("Alternatives to bingeing never work for me. I give up"), which are frequently characterized by *discounting positives, judgment focus, fortune telling,* and *dichotomous thinking.* The therapist and patient can review how the patient learned any other skill (e.g., riding a bike) and how she experienced gains and setbacks during the long process. The therapist should normalize difficulties in learning new skills and behaviors in treatment, and use this opportunity to reinforce successive approximations toward compliance.

Paradoxical Interventions

Rather than challenge resistance directly, the therapist can often promote compliance by diffusing any power struggle between patient and therapist. The use of paradoxical interventions, in which the patient is instructed to act opposite of what the treatment requires, may be one way to reduce resistance. Paradoxical interventions are particularly useful for general homework noncompliance. Instead of reassigning the homework as before, the therapist may ponder aloud whether the assignment was too difficult for the patient at this stage. The therapist essentially takes responsibility for giving the patient too much, rather than faulting the patient for her noncompliance. The therapist then asks the patient to do a lesser version over the coming week, perhaps one day of food records rather than all seven. The therapist emphasizes that the patient should do no more. It is important that this be done completely free of sarcasm or judgment. Often the patient will find the lower intensity assignment to be rather easy to fulfill, and will then go on to complete more than is required. The advantage of the paradoxical intervention is that, whatever the level of completion over the following week, it is in line with treatment recommendations, the therapist and patient are realigned, and the patient's compliance can be reinforced.

Adjusting Perfectionistic Expectations

Roadblocks often occur in treatment when the patient has a real or perceived setback that conflicts with her high expectations for herself and her progress. Identifying the patient's "should" statements and perfectionistic standards is the first step in altering her self-imposed expectations for success, treatment duration, a "cure," and never making mistakes. The patient may become frustrated with her slow progress, consider giving up on treatment, and catastrophize her chances of further improvement ("I will be your only patient who fails at treatment"). It is often useful to have the patient describe the feedback she would give to a friend who experienced a setback (*perspective taking, double-standard technique*) and to determine whether the same supportive, encouraging stance should apply to the patient's current struggles.

In all of the scenarios in which roadblocks occur, it is important that the therapist elicit the patient's concerns and difficulties with compliance, normalize her experience, and problem solve getting back on track.

To help prevent noncompliance and to underscore the importance of homework completion early in treatment, it is critical for the therapist to start each treatment session with a thorough review of the homework from the previous week. If the patient has not completed her homework, the therapist may choose to complete the assignment together in that session.

SAMPLE 20-SESSION TREATMENT PLAN

In this section, we present a detailed, session-by-session outline of the treatment for BN, an accessible overview of the more comprehensive treatment planning information presented throughout this book. For each session, suggested assessments and interventions are provided to help the clinician with treatment planning and report writing. This treatment plan outline is based on a 20-session treatment for BN or EDNOS, although it will require adaptation depending on each patient's idiosyncratic presentation, symptoms, comorbidity, and rate of treatment progress.

Intake Assessment

Assessment

- Thorough assessment of eating disorder symptoms (Form B.1 in Appendix B)
- Assessment of depression, anxiety, alcohol and substance abuse
- Review of patient's interpersonal and familial history, current and past body weights
- Assessment of suicidal risk (Form B.8 in Appendix B)
- Diagnosis (Table 1.1)
- Level-of-care decision making (Table 1.2, Figure 3.2)
- Case conceptualization (Form 3.2)

Session 1

Socialization to Treatment

- Inform patient of diagnosis
- Provide orientation to CBT for eating disorders (Figure 2.1)
- Provide patient with handout on eating disorders (Form 3.1)
- Collaboratively set treatment goals

Setting Up Multidisciplinary Treatment Team

- Referral to internist for blood work (ongoing as long as purging is present)
- Referral to psychiatrist and/or nutritionist, if warranted

Homework

- Complete Motivational Worksheet (Form 4.1)
- Begin bibliotherapy (suggestions included in Appendix C)

Session 2

Assessment

- Review homework (Form 4.1; assess reaction to self-help book)
- Evaluate presence and severity of eating disorder symptoms
- Assess motivation for treatment

Socialization to Treatment

- Psychoeducation about eating disorders

Behavioral Interventions

- Introduce the use of food records (Form 4.2)
- Begin weekly weighing
- Calculate BMI (Form B.6 in Appendix B)

Homework
- Complete Food Record daily (Form 4.2)

Session 3

Assessment
- Review daily food records thoroughly
- Evaluate presence and severity of eating disorder symptoms
- Assess motivation for treatment

Behavioral Interventions
- Discuss consequences of purging (Form 4.3)
- Set goal to immediately discontinue (or delay) purging
- Problem solve strategies to prevent purging behaviors
- Introduce regular, planned meals and snacks (Figure 4.2)

Homework
- Complete daily food records
- Discontinue (or delay) purging
- Adopt a regular, planned eating pattern

Session 4

Assessment
- Review homework
- Review of daily food records
- Evaluate presence and severity of eating disorder symptoms
- Assess motivation for treatment

Behavioral Interventions
- Conduct a functional analysis of binge triggers
- Introduce stimulus control interventions to decrease binge triggers (Form 4.4)

Homework
- Complete daily food records
- Practice stimulus control measures

Session 5

Assessment
- As in Session 4

Behavioral Interventions

- Introduce and practice "urge surfing"
- Brainstorm alternatives to bingeing (Forms 4.5 and 4.6)

Homework

- Complete daily food records
- Practice "urge surfing"
- Create list of chosen alternative coping strategies

Session 6

Assessment

- As in Session 4

Behavioral Interventions

- Introduce three steps to problem solving for likely binge situations
- Introduce and practice diaphragmatic breathing (Form 4.7)

Homework

- Complete daily food records
- Practice problem solving for upcoming binge situations
- Practice diaphragmatic breathing daily

Session 7

Assessment

- Review homework
- Review daily food records
- Review treatment progress to date
- Review use of behavioral interventions
- Problem solve any treatment setbacks

Session 8

Assessment

- As in Session 4

Cognitive Interventions

- Explain the thought–behavior connection

- Begin identifying cognitive distortions and automatic thoughts (Forms 4.8 and 4.10)
- Introduce and practice the A-B-C-D technique (Form 4.9)

Homework

- Complete daily food records
- Practice A-B-C-D technique to identify automatic thoughts (Form 4.9)

Session 9

Assessment

- As in Session 4

Cognitive Interventions

- Identify patterns in automatic thoughts
- Introduce cognitive restructuring techniques (Form 4.11)

Homework

- Complete daily food records
- Practice cognitive restructuring using Form 4.11

Session 10

Assessment

- As in Session 4

Cognitive Interventions

- Practice cognitive restructuring
- Generate list of food rules (Form 4.12)
- Discuss the advantages and disadvantages of food rules

Homework

- Complete daily food records
- Practice cognitive restructuring using Form 4.11
- Complete Food Rules Worksheet (Form 4.12)

Session 11

Assessment

- As in Session 4

Cognitive Interventions

- Practice cognitive restructuring
- Introduce and plan ahead to relax food rules

Homework

- Complete daily food records
- Experiment with relaxing food rules and reincorporating restricted foods

Session 12

Assessment

- As in Session 4

Cognitive Interventions

- Continue to plan for relaxing dietary rules and reintroducing restricted foods

Homework

- Complete daily food records
- Experiment with relaxing food rules and reincorporating restricted foods

Session 13

Assessment

- As in Session 4

Cognitive Interventions

- Continue to plan for relaxing dietary rules and reintroducing restricted foods
- Begin identifying perfectionistic standards
- Evaluate costs and benefits of holding perfectionistic standards
- Begin challenging perfectionistic standards using cognitive restructuring

Homework

- Complete daily food records
- Experiment with relaxing food rules and reincorporating restricted foods
- Practice identifying and challenging perfectionistic standards (Form 4.11)
- Complete Body Image Checklist (Form B.4 in Appendix B)

Session 14

Assessment

- As in Session 4

Cognitive Interventions

- Challenge perfectionistic beliefs using cognitive restructuring
- Introduce the double-standard technique, zero-point comparisons, and behavioral experiments (Form 4.13)

Body Image Interventions

- Redefine healthy (Table 4.1)
- Discuss the subjective nature of body image
- Identify body-checking and avoidance behaviors using Body Image Checklist (Form B.4 in Appendix B)
- Discuss progressive discontinuation of checking/avoidance behaviors

Homework

- Complete daily food records
- Challenge perfectionistic standards
- Record body image triggers
- Begin progressive discontinuation of checking/avoidance behaviors

Session 15

Assessment

- As in Session 4

Body Image Interventions

- Introduce cognitive restructuring for body image-related thoughts (Form 4.11)
- Challenge unrealistic standards for body and appearance
- Identify costs of the "perfect body" (Form 4.14)
- Introduce pie chart exercise (Form 4.15)

Homework

- Complete daily food records
- Continue reducing body-checking/avoidance behaviors
- Practice cognitive restructuring for body image-related thoughts
- Complete pie chart exercise (Form 4.15)

Session 16

Assessment

- As in Session 4

Body Image Interventions

- Complete reviewing history exercise
- Discuss patient's use of unfair comparisons and strategies to stop them
- Practice cognitive restructuring for body image-related thoughts, especially unfair comparisons (Form 4.11)

Homework

- Complete daily food records
- Use pie chart exercise to select one non-appearance-related task daily
- Practice cognitive restructuring for body image-related thoughts

Session 17

Assessment

- As in Session 4

Body Image Interventions

- Introduce positive data log

Supplementary Interventions

- Evaluate interpersonal difficulties
- Use interpersonal interventions and problem solving, as needed
- Use emotion regulation interventions, as needed

Homework

- Complete daily food records
- Complete positive data log daily
- Practice interpersonal problem solving or emotion regulation skills, as needed

Session 18

Assessment

- As in Session 4

Supplementary Interventions

- Use additional cognitive restructuring, as needed
- Continue interpersonal interventions, as needed
- Continue emotion regulation interventions, as needed

Homework

- Complete daily food records
- Practice interpersonal problem solving or emotion regulation skills, as needed

Session 19

Assessment

- As in Session 4

Relapse Prevention Interventions

- Review useful treatment interventions
- Identify past triggers for eating disorder symptoms
- Introduce the Relapse Roadmap (Form 4.17)

Homework

- Complete daily food records
- List past triggers and vulnerabilities to relapse

Session 20

Assessment

- As in Session 4

Relapse Prevention Interventions

- Continue to identify past triggers and likely vulnerabilities to relapse
- Complete Relapse Roadmap (Form 4.17)
- Differentiate "lapse" from "relapse"
- Conclude with termination

FORM 4.1. Motivation Worksheet

	Advantages of dieting, bingeing, and purging	Disadvantages of dieting, bingeing, and purging
Now		
In 5 years		

FORM 4.2. Food Record

Planning Ahead:

Day: M T W Th F Sa Su

Date: _____

Time	Location	Food/Drink Consumed	★	V/L	Emotions/Triggers/ Urges/Satisfaction

FORM 4.3.   Information for Patients about Purging

People with bulimia nervosa typically purge after binges and/or meals to lower their anxiety, to feel less bloated, and to reduce the number of calories absorbed by their bodies. Vomiting is the typical means of purging, but laxative use also is relatively common. Although vomiting or laxatives may reduce your discomfort in the short term, you most likely feel intense shame, disgust, and anxiety soon after purging. Purging also keeps the eating disorder cycle going, making it even more likely that you'll restrict and binge again in the future. You probably are aware that vomiting and laxative use are dangerous. What you may not know is that **purging is an ineffective way to lose weight.** This handout will explain why purging is ineffective, the potential medical consequences of purging, and how to stop.

IS PURGING DANGEROUS?

There are many medical and psychological consequences of purging, some of which can be fatal. Even irregular vomiting or laxative use can cause *dehydration*, which in turn can cause *organ damage*. Both vomiting and laxative use can lead to *electrolyte abnormalities*, which are changes in your body's levels of potassium, sodium, and chloride. An electrolyte imbalance is very serious and can lead to fatal *cardiac problems*. Purging can increase your risk for *dental erosion*, *periodontal disease*, *irritable bowel syndrome*, other gastrointestinal distress, and *osteoporosis*. Do not be lured into a false sense of safety because laxatives are available over the counter. Frequent use of laxatives can cause *intestinal damage*, *chronic constipation*, and *bowel tumors*. Frequent vomiting can cause *esophageal damage*, which can be fatal.

WHY IS VOMITING INEFFECTIVE?

Although most patients find this hard to believe at first, vomiting does not prevent your body from absorbing most of the calories ingested. Your body begins digesting food as soon as it is consumed, so calories are absorbed before you vomit. It also is impossible to vomit all food consumed; some of it will remain in your stomach afterward. Research has found that, on average, bulimic patients retain more than 53% of the calories from a binge. Often, they absorb much more than 50% of the calories consumed despite vomiting. You may believe that you have special "techniques" to increase the effectiveness of your vomiting, but these too are ineffective and dangerous. "Flushing," sustained vomiting, and use of "marker foods" do not work and may increase your risk for electrolyte imbalance and other medical consequences.

WHY ARE LAXATIVES INEFFECTIVE?

There are two basic kinds of laxatives: stimulant laxatives (Correctol, Senekot, Dulcolax, ex-lax) and bulking agents (Metamucil, Citrucel, FiberCon). Although they operate in different ways, neither decreases the amount of calories absorbed by the body. Laxatives only affect waste in your lower intestine, which is food that has already been fully digested by your body. Any weight lost after using laxatives is due to water loss, and this contributes to the serious risks of dehydration and electrolyte imbalance. Although you may feel less bloated after using laxatives, this sensation is temporary.

(cont.)

HOW CAN I STOP?

• *You should stop vomiting and using laxatives immediately.* It may feel difficult to stop purging abruptly, but it is possible and is the best way. Most people actually find it quite possible to stop vomiting and laxative use immediately. Stopping abruptly is preferred to gradual discontinuation of purging because the latter simply will prolong laxative withdrawal and anxiety symptoms.

• If you try but are unable to stop "cold turkey," then gradually increase the time between your binge and purge. Start by waiting 10 minutes after bingeing/eating, do something to distract yourself while waiting, and then see if the urge to purge remains. On each successive occasion, increase the amount of time you wait to purge. This method will help you learn to tolerate the anxiety, and eventually you will see for yourself that you do not need to purge in order for the anxiety and bloated feeling to subside.

• To make it easier to resist the urge to purge, remind yourself that this behavior is ineffective, read over the medical consequences of purging, throw out your supply of laxatives, and engage in a distracting activity after you eat (e.g., go for a walk, call a friend). The urge will pass—it always does!

WHAT CAN I EXPECT WHEN I STOP PURGING?

• When you initially stop vomiting after binges, you likely will feel intensely anxious, worried about weight gain, physically full and bloated, and unable to concentrate on other activities. These sensations may last a few minutes, a few hours, or, infrequently, a couple of days. As with all physical and mental sensations, these will pass on their own—you do not need to purge to get rid of these feelings. Each time you successfully resist the urge to vomit, it will get easier.

• When you stop relying on laxatives after binges, you will likely feel the same sensations as when you discontinue vomiting: anxiety, worry about weight gain, physically full and bloated, and difficulty concentrating on other activities. You also will likely feel constipated for several days and may gain a small amount of weight temporarily. If you have used laxatives frequently and for a long period of time, your lower intestine may be damaged and your body may be reliant on laxatives to produce a bowel movement. In these extreme cases, you may experience constipation for up to a few weeks. (See your medical doctor, who can discuss your options with you.)

• To help ease constipation without the use of stimulant, bulking, or herbal laxatives:

  • Eat regularly throughout the day, especially breakfast.
  • Drink more water.
  • Eat more whole grains, beans, fruits, and vegetables.
  • Engage in a moderate amount of exercise to stimulate your muscles.

FORM 4.4. 10 Steps to Stimulus Control

1. Access and availability.

2. Plan ahead.

3. Serve portions.

4. Out of sight, out of mind.

5. Routine, routine, routine.

6. Slow down.

7. Mindful eating.

8. Write it down.

9. Move!

10. "5-minute rule."

FORM 4.5. Alternative Coping Strategies

Binge trigger	Non-food alternative
👎 _____ _____	👍 _____ _____
👎 _____ _____	👍 _____ _____
👎 _____ _____	👍 _____ _____
👎 _____ _____	👍 _____ _____
👎 _____ _____	👍 _____ _____
👎 _____ _____	👍 _____ _____
👎 _____ _____	👍 _____ _____

FORM 4.6. Checklist of Possible Alternative Coping Strategies

Instructions: The following is a list of sample activities that may be effective for riding out urges to binge–purge, to calm yourself during times of stress, and to soothe emotional upset. The ideal activity requires concentration and is incompatible with eating. Check any that appeal to you.

☐ Go for a walk	☐ Stretch
☐ Call a friend	☐ Pray
☐ Engage in deep breathing	☐ Play a musical instrument
☐ Play a board game	☐ Make a gratitude list
☐ Read a novel	☐ Engage in scrapbooking
☐ Do yoga	☐ Read a magazine
☐ Clean a closet	☐ Write a letter
☐ Give yourself a manicure/pedicure	☐ Play with dog or cat
☐ Take a shower	☐ Do a crossword puzzle
☐ Relax in a park	☐ Dance
☐ Play with kids	☐ Get a massage
☐ Brush teeth	☐ Work in the garden
☐ Window shop	☐ Take a short nap
☐ Listen to music	☐ Visualize a relaxing place
☐ Knit	☐ Do a thought record
☐ Have a cup of tea	☐ Watch a favorite movie
☐ Exercise	☐ Arrange flowers
☐ Take a bubble bath	☐ Run an errand
☐ _____	☐ _____
☐ _____	☐ _____

FORM 4.7. Instructions for Diaphragmatic Breathing

To practice deep breathing, simply sit comfortably with your legs uncrossed, your hands in your lap or at your sides. Set a timer for a minimum of 5 minutes to alert you when you have finished this exercise. Work up to doing 20- to 30-minute sessions of diaphragmatic breathing.

Let your head fall back and, if you feel comfortable, close your eyes. You may also fix your eyes on one point in the room. Take several breaths as normal. Now direct your attention to your breath, noticing the sensations as you inhale and as you exhale. If you find that your mind wanders during this exercise, simply redirect your attention back to your breath.

Now place one hand on your abdomen, just below your rib cage. This hand should rise and fall with each breath. Breathe in slowly through your nose, allowing the air to travel deep into your body, then circling back out slowly, exhaling from your mouth. With each breath, concentrate on breathing more slowly and more deeply. You may intentionally push out your abdomen to make more room for your breath. Breathe in slowly, counting to 5. Inhaling for 1-2-3-4-5. Now slowly exhale, also counting to 5. Exhaling for 1-2-3-4-5. Continue breathing deeply, counting along with your breath. Breathe in for 1-2-3-4-5. Breathe out for 1-2-3-4-5.

There is no right or wrong way to breathe, simply try to keep your mind focused on your breath. Try to make each breath slower and deeper than the last. You might imagine breathing in fresh, clean air each time you inhale and, as you exhale, breathing out any tension or stress. Without judgment, notice any tension or discomfort in your body. Allow your breath to relax your body and your mind. Continue to slowly breathe in and out. Breathe in for 1-2-3-4-5. Breathe out for 1-2-3-4-5. When your alarm sounds, take several more slow, deep breaths, still keeping your mind focused on your breathing. Now, when you are ready, you may open your eyes.

FORM 4.8. Categories of Distorted Automatic Thoughts: A Guide for Patients

1. **Mind reading:** You assume that you know what people think without having sufficient evidence of their thoughts. "He thinks I'm a loser."

2. **Fortunetelling:** You predict the future negatively: Things will get worse, or there is danger ahead. "I'll fail that exam" or "I won't get the job."

3. **Catastrophizing:** You believe that what has happened or will happen will be so awful and unbearable that you won't be able to stand it. "It would be terrible if I failed."

4. **Labeling:** You assign global negative traits to yourself and others. "I'm undesirable" or "He's a rotten person."

5. **Discounting positives:** You claim that the positive things you or others do are trivial. "That's what husbands are supposed to do—so it doesn't count when he's nice to me" or "Those successes were easy, so they don't matter."

6. **Negative filter:** You focus almost exclusively on the negatives and seldom notice the positives. "Look at all of the people who don't like me."

7. **Overgeneralizing:** You perceive a global pattern of negatives on the basis of a single incident. "This generally happens to me. I seem to fail at a lot of things."

8. **Dichotomous thinking:** You view events or people in all-or-nothing terms. "I get rejected by everyone" or "It was a complete waste of time."

9. **Shoulds:** You interpret events in terms of how things should be rather than simply focusing on what is. "I should do well. If I don't, then I'm a failure."

10. **Personalizing:** You attribute a disproportionate amount of the blame to yourself for negative events, and you fail to see that certain events are also caused by others. "The marriage ended because I failed."

11. **Blaming:** You focus on the other person as the *source of* your negative feelings, and you refuse to take responsibility for changing yourself. "She's to blame for the way I feel now" or "My parents caused all my problems."

12. **Unfair comparisons:** You interpret events in terms of standards that are unrealistic—for example, you focus primarily on others who do better than you and find yourself inferior in the comparison. "She's more successful than I am" or "Others did better than I did on the test."

13. **Regret orientation:** You focus on the idea that you could have done better in the past rather than on what you can do better now. "I could have had a better job if I had tried" or "I shouldn't have said that."

14. **What if?:** You keep asking a series of questions about "what if" something happens, and you fail to be satisfied with any of the answers. "Yeah, but what if I get anxious?" or "What if I can't catch my breath?"

15. **Emotional reasoning:** You let your feelings guide your interpretation of reality. "I feel depressed; therefore, my marriage is not working out."

16. **Inability to disconfirm:** You reject any evidence or arguments that might contradict your negative thoughts. For example, when you have the thought "I'm unlovable," you reject as *irrelevant* any evidence that people like you. Consequently, your thought cannot be refuted. "That's not the real issue. There are deeper problems. There are other factors."

17. **Judgment focus:** You view yourself, others, and events in terms of evaluations as good–bad or superior–inferior rather than simply describing, accepting, or understanding. You continually measure yourself and others according to arbitrary standards and find that you and others fall short. You are focused on the judgments of others as well as your own judgments of yourself. "I didn't perform well in college," "If I take up tennis, I won't do well," or "Look how successful she is. I'm not successful."

Source: Leahy, Holland, and McGinn (2012).

FORM 4.9. A–B–C–D Technique

Activating Event (situation)	**Beliefs** (automatic thoughts)	**Consequences** (emotions and behaviors)	**Distortions** (biases in thinking)

FORM 4.10. Labeling the Distortion

Negative Automatic Thoughts	Associated Cognitive Distortions
"Skipping a meal means I am in control and better than others."	Overgeneralizing, "shoulds," emotional reasoning, judgment focus
"If I eat throughout the day, I will gain weight."	Fortunetelling, catastrophizing
"I am fat and unattractive."	Mind reading, labeling, dichotomous thinking, emotional reasoning, judgment focus
"I should be able to fit into smaller jeans."	"Shoulds," judgment focus
"If I don't purge after this meal, I will feel bloated for days and will be unable to concentrate at work."	Fortunetelling, catastrophizing, negative filter, dichotomous thinking
"My parents don't appreciate how hard I work."	Mind reading, negative filter, blaming
"This urge will last forever."	Fortunetelling, catastrophizing
"I know there will be a lot of food at the party tonight. I should eat less today so it doesn't ruin my whole week."	Catastrophizing, overgeneralizing, "shoulds"
"I can't skip a day at the gym. Otherwise, I will gain weight and feel terrible."	Fortunetelling, catastrophizing, dichotomous thinking, "shoulds"
"If I eat in front of my friends, they will think I am a pig."	Mind reading, labeling, dichotomous thinking, judgment focus
"My husband must think I am so weak and crazy."	Mind reading, labeling, negative filter, dichotomous thinking, judgment focus
"I feel so full. I ate too much. I feel like I've gained weight already."	Regret orientation, emotional reasoning
"Sweets are the only thing that will make me feel better."	Fortunetelling, discounting positives, dichotomous thinking
"Potato chips are a bad food. They are totally off limits."	Labeling, dichotomous thinking, judgment focus

FORM 4.11. Automatic Thought Record

Activating Event (situation)	**B**eliefs (automatic thoughts)	**C**onsequences (emotions)	Distortions	Evidence Supporting Thought	Evidence against Thought	Rational, Balanced Response
With whom? What? When? Where?	*What did I think/ imagine during the situation? What does this say about me? What does this say about my future? What do others think?*	*What did I feel in this situation? Sad, mad, happy, disappointed, guilty, ashamed, angry, frustrated, depressed, anxious, afraid, jealous?*	*Circle distortions evident in negative automatic thought* Mindreading Fortunetelling Catastrophizing Labeling Discounting positives Negative filter Overgeneralizing Dichotomous thinking Shoulds Personalizing Blaming Unfair comparisons Regret orientation What if? Emotional reasoning Inability to disconfirm Judgment focus	*Concrete, objective, observable facts*		*Rewrite your original thought to better reflect the evidence*

FORM 4.12. Food Rules Worksheet

Avoided, Restricted, and Feared Foods and Situations	Rank
Example: *Eating multiple foods in one sitting*	3
Example: *potato chips*	5

Rank

0———1———2———3———4———5

Least avoidance   Most avoidance

FORM 4.13. Zero-Point Comparisons: Learn to Stop Your Upward Comparisons

Quality being rated: _____

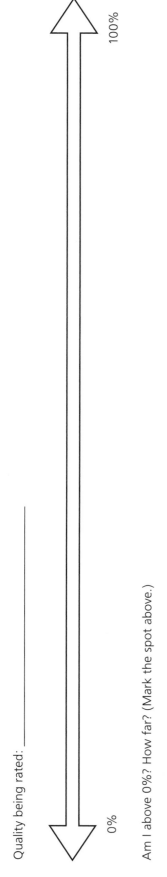

0%

100%

Am I above 0%? How far? (Mark the spot above.)

Define 0%	For what qualities or successes can I give myself credit?

FORM 4.14. Costs of the "Perfect" Body

Describe the "Perfect" Body	Costs of Attaining the "Perfect" Body

FORM 4.15. Self-Image Worksheet

How I saw myself at the beginning of treatment. What was most important to me? How did I evaluate myself?

How I would like to see myself. What areas of my life are improved? What else is important to me? Where would I like to invest more time?

FORM 4.16. Coping Cards

COPING CARD

Problematic Situation:

Possible Coping Responses:

-

-

-

-

-

COPING CARD

Problematic Situation:

Possible Coping Responses:

-

-

-

-

-

FORM 4.17. Relapse Roadmap

Bumps in the Road (trigger situations and early signs of relapse)	**Detours from Recovery** (risky responses)	**Seatbelts and Airbags** (healthier, safer alternatives)
Example: • *Gain 5 pounds and feel fat*	*Example:* • *Start a strict diet* • *Skip lunch* • *Pinch fat in mirror* • *Feel hopeless and binge*	*Example:* • *Regular, moderate eating* • *Resume food records* • *Review pie chart* • *Stimulus control and challenge hopeless thoughts*

CHAPTER 5

Case Example

SESSION 1

Presenting Problem

Jenna was a 26-year-old newlywed who presented for treatment after more than 6 years of bingeing and purging. She had no prior psychological or psychiatric treatment. For the 2 years prior to intake, since completing business school, she was employed at a prestigious firm in her "dream job." At intake, Jenna reported concern about the effect her eating disorder was having on her concentration at work, prompting her to seek treatment. She reported that thoughts of food, her appearance, and her weight consumed nearly all her mental energy. She was also concerned about trust issues and the impact her eating disorder was having on her relationship with her husband, from whom she kept her bingeing and purging secret. Jenna and her husband were planning to start a family in the coming year, and Jenna reported concern about purging during pregnancy, handling pregnancy weight gain, and being a good role model as a mother.

Intake assessment

Symptoms of Bulimia Nervosa

Jenna started bingeing and purging 6 years prior to intake following a 6-month period of strict dieting and significant weight loss. The frequency of bingeing and purging increased over the years and, at the time of intake, occurred approximately twice daily. During a typical day, Jenna reported that she ate a piece of fruit for breakfast, a small salad (no dressing) with grilled chicken and broccoli as a late lunch, and a small platter of assorted sushi for dinner. She tried not to eat in between meals and believed that doing so is a sign of "weakness." Her diet was not at all varied, and these were the only foods she considered "safe" to eat. Jenna occasionally vomited after a meal if she ate a "bad food" or a portion she considered "excessive." Almost every evening, while working late, Jenna binged at her desk. Tempting binge foods were readily available in her office kitchen. A typical binge was 15 cookies, a handful of potato chips, and 10 miniature candy bars. Jenna reported that she "hid" in

Assessment of BN symptoms

This case example is completely fictionalized. While the descriptions of symptoms and interventions are based on Rene Zweig's experience working with many patients, the case material presented here does not reflect a real case.

her office while bingeing. She ate the food very rapidly, felt out of control, and subsequently felt ashamed and bloated. She then immediately vomited to ease her guilt and physical discomfort.

At 5'4" and 110 pounds, Jenna's BMI at intake was 19, indicating that she was borderline underweight. Her highest adult weight was 140 pounds, which immediately preceded her strict diet 6 years ago. Her lowest adult weight was 103 pounds 2 years earlier when she was exercising intensely. Jenna's scores were highly elevated on the Restraint, Eating Concern, and Shape Concern subscales of the EDE-Q. At intake, Jenna reported strong motivation to discontinue bingeing and purging, although she felt her current diet was otherwise healthy. She described feeling unattractive and "too flabby" at her current weight, and she was intensely afraid of weight gain.

Assessment of Comorbid Conditions

Jenna reported feeling significant anxiety most days, characterized by worry about the future, work, and her relationship. Her Beck Anxiety Inventory (BAI) score was high (27) at intake. She exhibited no compulsive behaviors and denied experiencing panic attacks. She denied depressive symptoms and any past depressive episodes. Her BDI score

Assessment of depression, anxiety, alcohol use, and substance abuse

was low (5). She denied any current or past substance abuse, and she reported drinking only occasionally. At intake, Jenna disclosed that she is quite regimented in her routines, in completing tasks, and in organization and cleanliness. She reported having difficulty being flexible when collaborating with others on team projects. She also found it difficult to relax until all of her work was complete. The SCID-II confirmed that Jenna met diagnostic criteria for obsessive–compulsive personality disorder. Jenna reported having a fulfilling and supportive relationship with her husband, and her Dyadic Adjustment Scale score was in the satisfied range (109). Jenna's diagnoses include:

Axis I: Bulimia nervosa (307.51); generalized anxiety disorder (300.02)   *Diagnosis*
Axis II: Obsessive–compulsive personality disorder (301.4)
Axis III: Slightly underweight; no other medical conditions reported
Axis IV: Stressors related to employment, recent marriage, family, recent move, and
           reduced social support network
Axis V: Current: GAF = 55
           Highest past year: GAF = 55

Evaluation of Suicide Risk

Jenna reported significant frustration with her eating disorder and worried about how it would affect her future. However, she reported feeling otherwise hopeful and denied any suicidal thoughts or intent. Jenna denied any past

Assessment of suicidal risk

suicidal attempts or gestures. She reported no familial history of mood disorders or suicidality.

Psychotropic Medications

Jenna had never seen a psychiatrist or been prescribed psychotropic medication. She was open to the idea of medications to improve her anxiety and eating disorder.

Socialization to Treatment

During the initial session, the therapist described the cognitive-behavioral model for BN to Jenna, showing how her obsession with her weight and shape set off a desire to diet, to carefully control her food intake, and to deprive herself of seemingly "bad" foods. This ongoing pattern of dietary restriction, hypervigilence about food choices, and strict food rules led to deprivation and hunger. The deprivation and hunger, when combined with an emotional trigger and/or the accessibility of "trigger" foods, immediately precipitated a binge. Jenna related well to this model and recognized having feelings of guilt and disgust following a binge. Her inability to tolerate physical discomfort and negative affect, combined with a fear of weight gain following the binge, triggered vomiting. Jenna also recognized that she would then vow to be "good" the following morning, which included resuming her strict dietary control and perfectionistic standards (see Figure 5.1). The therapist recommended that Jenna begin reading *Overcoming Binge Eating* by Christopher Fairburn to better understand BN, and also provided Jenna with a copy of the Information for Patients about Bulimia Nervosa (Form 3.1).

Orientation to CBT for BN

Case conceptualization

Jenna and the therapist discussed the potential medical consequences of BN, particularly purging. The therapist requested that Jenna see her physician as soon as possible for blood work to assess for electrolyte imbalance. The therapist also requested that Jenna schedule a consultation for a psychotropic medication evaluation and provided her with psychiatric referrals.

Referral to internist

Referral to psychiatrist

At the end of the initial session, the therapist asked Jenna to describe her goals for treatment, ensuring that her treatment goals were realistic and well defined:

Set treatment goals

1. Stop bingeing and purging.
2. Become less obsessive about food.
3. Improve body image.
4. Learn to exercise moderately.
5. Learn to better manage anxiety and stress.

In light of the cognitive-behavioral model of BN, the therapist suggested Jenna add the following to her treatment goals:

6. Reduce dietary restriction.
7. Modify perfectionistic beliefs.
8. Improve work performance and concentration.

SESSION 2

As with all subsequent sessions, the therapist began the second session by setting a collaborative agenda with the patient:

Set session agenda

Cognitive Factors:
(perfectionism, dichotomous thinking,
overemphasis on weight/shape)
- *Constant attention to own shape, weight, & food*
- *Intensely afraid of weight gain*
- *"I am only lovable if I am thin and perfect"*
- *"If I relinquish control, I'll binge wildly"*
- *Holds dichotomous beliefs about self & others*
- *Vows to be "good" after bingeing*
- *"Eating less than others proves I am in control"*

Restrictive Behaviors:
(food rules, restrictive dieting, forbidden foods)
- *Restricted food intake*
- *Views snacking as a sign of "weakness"*
- *Avoids all fats, red meat, snack foods, and dessert*
- *Eats small portions at each meal and often skips meals*
- *Has very few "safe" foods in diet*

Body Image:
(checking, avoidance, distortions,
negative beliefs)
- *Feels "flabby" despite low body weight*
- *"I am unattractive"*
- *Feels bloated and "fat" after any unplanned snacking or a binge*
- *Weighs self multiple times daily*
- *Frequent pinching of body fat, checking self in mirror, and trying on "skinny" clothes*

Situational Triggers:
(hunger, deprivation, social, environmental)

- *Works late most nights*
- *Hungry in evenings after restricting food intake all day*
- *"Forbidden" foods are readily available in her office*

Compensatory Behaviors:

- *Vomits after all binge episodes*
- *Occasionally vomits after large meals or after consuming "bad" foods*
- *Purging temporarily reduces anxiety*

Emotional Triggers:

- *High anxiety most days*
- *Loneliness*
- *Work-related stressors*
- *Exhaustion*
- *Feeling overwhelmed*

Bingeing:

- *Binges 2x daily currently*
- *Has been bingeing for past 6 years*

FIGURE 5.1. Completed Case Conceptualization Worksheet for Jenna.

1. Address Jenna's comments and questions following the initial session.
2. Review homework: Review Jenna's reactions to *Overcoming Binge Eating*; follow up on psychiatric consultation; follow up on prescribed blood tests.
3. Begin weekly weighing.
4. Treatment motivation.
5. Introduce first steps for behavioral change.
6. Assign homework and summarize session interventions.

At the start of the second session, Jenna vocalized several questions and concerns she had following the intake session. The therapist addressed Jenna's questions, and together they discussed the effectiveness of cognitive-behavioral treatment, the importance of addressing the dietary restriction to fully treat the bingeing–purging, and her fears of dramatic weight gain. Although scary for her, it was expected that Jenna would gain some weight during treatment in order to obtain a healthy body weight. The therapist and Jenna discussed how they would later work together to improve her body image at her new, healthy weight.

Jenna relayed that she read the first three chapters of *Overcoming Binge Eating*. She found the book to be informative and felt like "it read **Review homework** my mind." Jenna found comfort in not being alone in her bingeing behavior, and she felt more confident about treatment knowing that her problem was well understood. Jenna reported that she scheduled a psychiatric consultation and also made an appointment with her internist for that same week. The therapist thanked Jenna for completing all of the homework and informed her that continued compliance is a positive indicator of treatment success.

The therapist introduced weekly weighing, informing Jenna that once-weekly weigh-ins were the easiest and most reliable way to monitor weight. The weekly weighing provides objective information about any changes over the course of treatment and is more reliable and less obses- **Calculate BMI** **Weekly weighing** sive than Jenna's habit of weighing herself multiple times daily. The therapist noted that body weight tends to fluctuate as a result of water retention, sodium intake, and hormones, and thus these fluctuations do not reflect actual weight gain. Jenna recognized that her weight fluctuated significantly day to day and even within the same day, and she agreed not to weigh herself between sessions. The therapist suggested that Jenna hide her scale in her closet to reduce the temptation to weigh herself between sessions. After weighing Jenna in this session, the therapist then assisted her in calculating her BMI. Jenna was surprised to learn that, at a BMI of 19, she was considered marginally underweight. She also recognized that her body image has been persistently negative, even when she was significantly underweight (BMI = 17.5) 2 years earlier. Using the BMI table as a guide, Jenna saw that any weight between 116 and 140 pounds was considered healthy for her height. Although she again expressed concern about the possibility of weight gain, Jenna agreed to focus on her goal of treating the eating disorder and becoming healthier, while suspending efforts to control her weight as much as possible. The therapist reassured Jenna that uncontrolled weight gain is not only uncommon, but also is not the goal of treatment. Treatment would focus on helping Jenna become healthier and more flexible with food. In addition, the therapist and Jenna agreed that she could always return to her pretreatment weight control habits if she was truly unsatisfied with the results of treatment and the amount of weight gained. Thus, treatment itself was framed as an experiment, and Jenna felt more comfortable trusting the process knowing that she retained some control over her choices.

Although Jenna reported high motivation for change at the start of treatment, interventions to improve motivation are almost always warranted. The therapist asked Jenna to name

the advantages of engaging in treatment for her eating disorder, and the therapist recorded her responses on the Motivation Worksheet (Form 4.1): "healthier, more trust with my husband, stop bingeing, less obsessed with food and weight, better concentration at work, more accepting of my body, and able to get pregnant" (see Figure 5.2). Jenna also identified her fears of fully engaging in treatment, and these were recorded as current disadvantages on the worksheet: "a lot of effort, might fail, might gain weight, might become more obsessive, clothes won't fit, will feel self-conscious, and will get more anxious." The therapist then asked Jenna to consider what her life would look like in 5 years if she continued to binge, purge, and restrict, and the therapist recorded these advantages and disadvantages in their respective boxes on the worksheet: "stay thin and avoid anxiety"; "might be hospitalized, might lose my job, might jeopardize my marriage, will be

	Advantages of dieting, bingeing, and purging	Disadvantages of dieting, bingeing, and purging
Now	• *Prevents weight gain* • *Can wear smaller clothing size* • *Illusion of being in control* • *Don't have to face anxieties about change and fear of failure in treatment*	• *Unhealthy* • *Affects relationship with husband* • *Bingeing feels terrible and out of control* • *Constantly think about food, weight, & appearance* • *Difficulty concentrating at work* • *Vomiting is gross and uncomfortable* • *Have to lie to husband, family, and friends*
In 5 years	• *Stay thin* • *Avoid anxiety of weight gain*	• *Can't get pregnant/have a healthy pregnancy if dieting and purging* • *Would be too distracted and impatient to be a good mother* • *Would be a bad role model if I do have children* • *Might jeopardize my marriage* • *Could lose my job* • *Could be hospitalized* • *Disgusted with myself* • *Dental decay from vomiting* • *Might develop health problems from vomiting for so many years*

FIGURE 5.2. Completed Motivation Worksheet for Jenna.

unhealthy, will stay obsessed with food, would be a bad role model to my children, will still be bingeing and purging, and will be disgusted with myself." Jenna easily recognized that the advantages far outweighed the disadvantages and her fears of recovery.

Jenna was then ready to begin the behavioral change portion of treatment, and the therapist explained that Jenna should begin record-

Daily food records

ing her food intake over the coming week. Food records would keep her aware of her decisions in the moment, are a key component of effective treatment, and would be particularly useful in identifying patterns and triggers for her bingeing. Jenna agreed, although she cited concerns that paying close attention to her food intake would increase her obsessive thoughts, make her anxious, and increase the frequency of her binges. The therapist assured Jenna that this is a normal concern, that this outcome is unusual, and that the coming week could be used as a test of her predictions. The therapist explained each of the food record columns to Jenna, and together they completed the sheet using her food intake from that day. The therapist asked Jenna to record all food and drink consumed every day, to note any binges and purges on the sheet, and to record any comments or emotional reactions to eating or choosing not to eat. The therapist also requested that Jenna make no changes to her diet over the coming week, but to eat as usual so together they could easily ascertain her starting point.

To close the session, Jenna and the therapist reviewed the points discussed, and the therapist reiterated the assigned homework: Jenna was to continue reading *Overcoming Binge Eating*, not weigh herself between sessions, and begin recording her food intake daily.

Recap session

Assign homework

SESSION 3

The therapist again started this session by setting a collaborative agenda, briefly reviewing Jenna's week, and checking on her home-

Thorough review of daily food records

work completion. The focus of the third session was to review Jenna's food records in detail, beginning to note eating patterns, binge-eating triggers, and periods of restriction. Jenna's eating remained similar to the patterns she described at intake. Her food records indicated that she ate very little food during the day, ate dinner at her desk while working, and typically binged soon after dinner (see Figure 5.3). Jenna also noted that she consistently felt "exhausted" and "overwhelmed" prior to her urges to binge. Thus, the therapist and Jenna noted that her binges were predictably triggered by strong negative emotion, boredom, fatigue, and sustained periods of deprivation. By the time she ate dinner, Jenna had eaten very little during the day and experienced both physical hunger and feelings of deprivation.

To address the periods of deprivation that contributed to Jenna's bingeing, the next step in behavioral change was introduced.

Regular, planned eating

A schedule of regular, evenly spaced meals and snacks was developed in session. The therapist explained that, by eating every 3 to 4 hours throughout the day, Jenna would experience less hunger and would, therefore, be less prone to bingeing in the evening. Eating throughout the day also would challenge one of Jenna's food rules, allowing her to see that relinquishing rigid control actually decreases bingeing. Just as she was instructed to make eating at the scheduled times a priority, Jenna also was instructed to not eat between scheduled times, thus allowing her to prac-

Day: M (T) W Th F Sa Su

Date: _November 30_

Time	Location	Food/Drink Consumed	*	V/L	Emotions/Triggers/ Urges/Satisfaction
7:30	Home— kitchen table	Bowl of blueberries Coffee w/ Splenda			Today is going to be a stressful day! Good, healthy breakfast
10 am	Desk	Coffee w/ Splenda			
1:15 pm	Desk	Small tossed mixed greens with chicken, cucumbers, tomatoes, & broccoli			Good lunch. Very full.
3:15	Desk	Seltzer—1 can			
5 pm	Conference room	Diet Coke			Tired. Irritable. Stressed.
7:30 pm	Desk	5 Peanut M&Ms			In stressful meeting. Couldn't resist. Feel so guilty. Should've waited until dinner.
8:45 pm	Desk	Sushi—4 pieces & 1 roll			So busy with work, barely noticed eating. Will be a late night :(
9 pm	Desk	Handful M&Ms	*		Boss just criticized my work. Angry. Lonely. Tired.
		Package peanut butter crackers Package Oreo cookies 3 more Oreos 2 handfuls mixed nuts 5 mini Reese's cups 2 chocolate donuts	* * * * * *	 V	Already blown it. Feel so fat. Shouldn't have eaten those M&Ms. Relief to vomit. I am a disgusting pig.

FIGURE 5.3. Completed Food Record for Jenna.

tice riding out urges to binge. Last, Jenna was to practice eating on schedule rather than listening to internal cues, which tend to be unreliable for patients at this stage of treatment. Jenna would relearn normal feelings of hunger/satiety over time. The therapist addressed Jenna's fears of weight gain and reviewed the cognitive-behavioral model, again highlighting the role of deprivation in bingeing.

The therapist also requested that Jenna commit not to vomit or use laxatives after meals or binges over the coming week. The thera- *Discontinue purging* pist explained that if she retained purging as an option, it would make bingeing more likely by sustaining the belief that the effects of binges can be reduced or eliminated. For most patients, purging also gives immediate anxiety relief following a binge, which further maintains the eating disorder cycle. Jenna was unsure whether she could adhere to this commitment, but she agreed to try. The therapist explained to Jenna that vomiting is ineffective for weight loss, as the research shows that fewer than 50% of calories ingested are purged. Jenna was skeptical about the truth of this statement, and she disclosed to her therapist that she used "special techniques" to ensure that all food was purged. The therapist provided Jenna with the Information for Patients about Purging handout (see Form 4.3), and together they discussed how digestion works, including that the stomach churns and mixes food. Thus, "marker" foods are ineffective because they are mixed with other foods—foods are not simply layered in the stomach and then vomited in reverse order. The therapist also explained that "flushing," drinking water while vomiting to completely empty the stomach, is particularly dangerous and can lead to cardiac arrest. The therapist further explained that laxatives are ineffective because they simply rid the body of food that has already been digested; thus, the calories have already been absorbed. Vomiting and laxative use are some of the most dangerous symptoms of BN and, because they are ineffective, should be stopped "cold turkey." Although most patients find it difficult to believe, a majority are able to discontinue all purging immediately (however, later lapses are also to be expected). The therapist explained that discontinued purging effectively disrupts the eating disorder cycle, and would likely immediately reduce the severity of binges. Jenna and her therapist discussed alternative ways to reduce anxiety following a binge to avert vomiting, including calling her husband, distracting herself by taking a walk, and doing deep-breathing exercises (see Form 4.6). The session again was closed with a review of interventions covered and homework assigned.

SESSIONS 4–7

Jenna arrived to the fourth treatment session excited that she had not binged at all the previous week. She described the eating schedule as "difficult" and "scary," but found she had less of a desire to binge after dinner because she had eaten more throughout the day. Jenna also relayed that recording her food intake kept her "aware" and motivated. As she had not binged since the last session, Jenna had no difficulty not purging. The therapist reinforced Jenna's rapid progress and noted that this was a positive sign for treatment. At the same time, the therapist noted that they needed to help Jenna develop coping strategies for urges that inevitably will arise in the future.

Over the next several sessions, Jenna and her therapist focused on *Functional analysis* preventing binge triggers, analyzing binges that occurred, and using *of binge triggers*

behavioral coping skills. The therapist and Jenna identified
and tested alternative behaviors she can use in response to
her most common binge triggers (see Figure 5.4). To address two of her common triggers, fatigue
and feeling overwhelmed, Jenna began taking a 5-minute walk after dinner as a break from work
and to decrease stress. Because a walk was sometimes not enough to reduce her tension, Jenna's
therapist also taught her to practice diaphragmatic breathing for
10 minutes. Jenna found this to be a relaxing and effective strat-
egy to get through urges to binge. Another common trigger was being alone, and Jenna found
several alternative strategies to bingeing when lonely: eating dinner with a colleague; calling her
husband if she had an urge to binge; listening to music while working in the evenings; and, if
necessary, going home to prevent being alone and isolated in the office. Seeing or being offered
tempting foods was also a common binge trigger. Although she was less vulnerable after eating
meals throughout the day and after eating a normal dinner, Jenna found that taking an alternate
route to the restroom helped her avoid seeing tempting foods in the office pantry. Jenna found
that completing her food records and practicing the stimulus control techniques decreased the frequency of binge urges, and she learned to effectively cope with most remaining urges.

The therapist also demonstrated urge surfing techniques for Jenna, helping
her to visualize the rapid onset, rising discomfort, and slow passing of urges.
Jenna learned that she did not need to give in to urges because they typically pass on their own
within 10 minutes, and she learned to use distraction techniques while waiting their passing.

Identify alternative activities

Diaphragmatic breathing

Stimulus control

Urge surfing

Binge trigger	Non-food alternative
👎 Fatigue	👍 Take a break from work
👎 Feeling overwhelmed	👍 5-minute walk after dinner
👎 Stress	👍 Diaphragmatic breathing
👎 Loneliness	👍 Call husband or a friend
👎 Presence of trigger foods	👍 Work from home instead of office
👎 Boredom	👍 Take alternate route to restroom to avoid pantry
	👍 Listen to music

FIGURE 5.4. Completed Alternative Coping Strategies for Jenna.

SESSIONS 8–10

As Jenna's eating pattern improved and she became more adept at using behavioral strategies to prevent binges, the focus of treatment shifted to cognitive interventions. Jenna and her therapist discussed

Explain the thought–behavior connection

how her interpretations of situations (her automatic thoughts) determined her behavioral and emotional reactions to those situations. Although Jenna had not binged in several weeks, she and her therapist discussed one of her past binge situations to identify the associated negative automatic thoughts (see Figure 5.5). When Jenna was working late in the evening, feeling bored, and still somewhat hungry after eating dinner, she

A-B-C-D technique

was likely to experience an urge to binge. Jenna recognized that she often thought, for example, "It is useless, I might as well binge"; "The urge will never go away unless I binge"; and "Eating just a few cookies now will cheer me up." Jenna recognized that when these automatic thoughts arose, she was more likely to feel hopeless, anxious, and frustrated. She was also much more likely to give in to the craving and then binge. Once Jenna gained experience riding out her urges to binge and using alternative behavioral coping strategies, she and her therapist were able to identify evidence inconsistent with those

Cognitive restructuring

automatic thoughts. Jenna's therapist guided her through completing an Automatic Thought Record in session (see Figure 5.6), together identifying more balanced, rational responses for that situation. The therapist explained that Jenna could complete a written thought record in a vulnerable moment to challenge the negative automatic thought. Jenna immediately recognized that this technique was useful for challenging many of her negative automatic thoughts across various situations. Jenna continued completing thought records between sessions whenever she felt depressed or significantly anxious or had a strong desire to restrict, binge, or purge. Jenna quickly saw a pattern in her typical distortions and automatic thoughts, and she learned not to act on these thoughts so readily.

Activating Event (situation)	**Beliefs** (automatic thoughts)	**Consequences** (emotions and behaviors)	**Distortions** (biases in thinking)
Working late in evening Bored and alone Hungry after a small dinner Presence of binge foods	"It is useless. I might as well binge now." "The urge will never go away unless I binge." "Eating just a few cookies now will cheer me up."	Hopeless Anxious Frustrated Binge	Fortunetelling Emotional reasoning Negative filter Inability to disconfirm Dichotomous thinking

FIGURE 5.5. Completed A-B-C-D Technique for Jenna.

Activating Event (situation)	Beliefs (automatic thoughts)	Consequences (emotions)	Distortions	Evidence Supporting Thought	Evidence against Thought	Rational, Balanced Response
With whom? What? When? Where?	What did I think/imagine during the situation? What does this say about me? What does this say about my future? What do others think?	What did I feel in this situation? Sad, mad, happy, disappointed, guilty, ashamed, angry, frustrated, depressed, anxious, afraid, jealous?	Circle distortions evident in negative automatic thought	Concrete, objective, observable facts		Rewrite your original thought to better reflect the evidence
Working late			Mindreading	I have binged many times in this situation	I have learned that urges last about 10 minutes	Urges feel like they last forever but really only last about 10 minutes
After dinner			(Fortunetelling)		Even though I had a strong urge, I have not purged on a few occasions in the past	
Still slightly hungry	"It is useless; I might as well binge."	Hopeless	Catastrophizing	I could easily choose to binge now		I can resist urges
Sitting at desk	"This urge will never go away unless I binge."	Anxious	Labeling		Calling my husband and doing deep breathing help me get through urges to binge	I can resist urges to binge by using my coping strategies
Alone	"Eating just a few cookies now will cheer me up."	Frustrated	(Discounting positives)			
Tired	"This job is so difficult and time consuming; I have nothing else in my life to make me happy."	Sad	Negative filter			It is difficult, but I always feel so much better when I resist the urge to binge
	"I am too weak."	Lonely	Overgeneralizing		I usually feel worse after a binge	
			Dichotomous thinking			
			Shoulds			
			Personalizing			
			Blaming			
			Unfair comparisons			
			Regret orientation			
			What if?			
			(Emotional reasoning)			
			(Inability to disconfirm)			
			(Judgment focus)			

FIGURE 5.6. Completed Automatic Thought Record for Jenna.

SESSIONS 10–13

During the first portion of session 10, Jenna and her therapist continued practicing cognitive restructuring techniques. Toward the latter part of session 10, the focus then shifted to addressing Jenna's food rules and lingering dietary restriction. As Jenna and her therapist worked on identifying and challenging her many negative automatic thoughts in the previous sessions, they together noticed how often she labeled particular foods as "bad," judged herself for eating in certain contexts, and compared her eating patterns with others' habits. To challenge Jenna's food rules and to reduce her dietary rigidity, Jenna and her therapist created a list of her "forbidden foods" and food rules (see Figure 5.7). This list included rules about the acceptable quantities and frequencies of meals, specific foods she did not allow herself to eat, foods she ate only in the context of a binge, and foods she ate but with significant discomfort and judgment. To create this list, the therapist and Jenna together reviewed all past food records, noting binge foods and the patterns and thoughts related to food intake. To identify other food rules, the therapist asked Jenna to record all foods she avoided or felt guilty about throughout the week. Jenna also walked through a grocery store, noting all foods she would describe as "bad" or "off limits." She added these foods to the list, rating each according to how much anxiety they created for her.

Identify food rules

Jenna and her therapist then discussed the advantages and disadvantages of keeping these foods off limits. Jenna recognized that avoiding these foods gave her the illusion of control and reduced her anxiety about bingeing but concurrently reinforced her all-or-nothing thinking about food. Her therapist noted that avoidance also contributed to thoughts that she had "blown it" after consuming even a small amount of these foods, thus likely triggering a binge. Jenna added that she only consumed these foods when bingeing, and it would be a relief and more enjoyable to have them in other contexts. Jenna further added that she would feel "normal" if she was able to be around these foods with less anxiety. Because Jenna saw the advantages of reincorporating these foods into her diet, the therapist explained how this would be accomplished slowly and under safe circumstances, thereby preventing bingeing.

For her first experience with eating a formerly restricted food, Jenna brought popcorn (a food she rated "3," or moderately anxiety provoking) into her 11th session. The therapist asked Jenna to make predictions about how much anxiety she would feel eating the popcorn, how long her anxiety would last, and what physical sensations she would experience. Jenna then ate the popcorn in session while the therapist instructed her to describe the tastes, the textures, and the experience. Jenna noted her anxiety levels throughout. After finishing the popcorn, Jenna again noted her anxiety levels. Although Jenna's anxiety increased while eating the popcorn, it did not remain significantly elevated as she predicted. She did report feeling some guilt and physical discomfort, although not as strongly as predicted. The therapist helped Jenna recognize the inaccuracy of her predictions about eating this food, and they then together challenged her negative thoughts such as, "This food is bad. I have lost control. I will be tempted to eat 'bad' foods for the rest of the day. I will certainly gain weight now." To end the session, Jenna and her therapist problem solved how to eat normally for the remainder of the day, adhering to her meal schedule and not putting herself into a binge situation. Jenna reported feeling calm and comfortable by the end of the session.

Reincorporate restricted foods

For homework over the next week and in the two subsequent sessions, Jenna was to rein-

Avoided, Restricted, and Feared Foods and Situations	Rank
Chicken	0
Vegetables	0
Tofu	0
Diet sodas	0
Sushi (no rice)	0
Fat-free, sugar-free yogurt	0
Fruits—apples, berries, and oranges	0
Bananas	1
Skim milk	1
Fat-free yogurt	1
Brown rice	1
Sushi with rice	1
Whole wheat pasta	2
Snacking between meals	2
Eating multiple foods in one meal	2
Juice	3
Popcorn	3
Pretzels	3
Eating full portions at meals	3
Potatoes	3
Licorice, gummy bears, or hard candies	4
Regular soda	4
Cheese	4
White pasta or rice	4
Sandwiches on whole grain bread	4
Cookies	5
Potato chips	5
Cakes	5
Hamburgers	5
Fried foods	5
Pizza	5
Mayonnaise	5
Peanut butter	5

FIGURE 5.7. Completed Food Rules Worksheet for Jenna.

corporate three restricted foods into her diet each week, slowly working up to the more difficult food options. Jenna was to plan a specific, safe time to eat the forbidden food, to have a limited quantity available, and to plan a non-food activity for immediately after the experiment. For example, Jenna decided it would be safe to experiment with restricted foods after her normal lunch, when she would not be too hungry and when she could then immediately occupy herself with work as a distraction technique. Jenna was compliant with this homework, and she found that it took about three experiments with each food before her anxiety diminished and she no longer worried about bingeing afterward. As she became more comfortable with reincorporating formerly restricted foods, Jenna noted that she also felt more comfortable resisting those foods in natural, unplanned situations. Jenna practiced saying to herself, "I now can trust myself to have these foods if I want them. I don't have to eat this just because it is here, and I don't have to binge on it to have it. I can have this later when the circumstances make it safer for me."

SESSIONS 13–14

Session 13 started with a continuation of expanding Jenna's diet, and the therapist then transitioned into interventions for perfectionism. Although Jenna had previously made significant progress in **Identify perfectionistic standards** learning to recognize, challenge, and modify her negative automatic thoughts, much of her thinking remained rigid and perfectionistic. Jenna still maintained noticeably high standards for herself in most areas of her life. She often felt anxious after making a single mistake, and she frequently felt like she was falling short of attainable standards. For example, despite being **Evaluate costs and benefits of perfectionistic standards** a compliant and responsive patient, she routinely commented that she should be doing better in therapy, apologized for not completing her homework perfectly, and felt quite demoralized after any setback with her eating disorder. Jenna also frequently described herself as a "bad" wife, employee, friend, and daughter. Jenna and her therapist discussed the ways in which her high standards contributed to her anxiety, interfered with her relationships, and decreased her feelings of self-worth. In sessions 13 and 14, and as homework in between, the therapist guided Jenna through several interventions to challenge her perfectionistic beliefs. Jenna found the double-standard technique and automatic thought records to be useful for putting her beliefs into perspective.

Zero-point comparisons was a particularly useful intervention for Jenna as it allowed her to acknowledge her imperfections while simultaneously giving herself credit for her accomplishments. Because Jenna had a tendency to **Challenge perfectionistic beliefs** declare herself a "complete failure" and routinely compared herself to perfection rather than attainable standards, the zero-point comparisons technique was an important tool to challenge these perfectionistic comparisons. The therapist explained the steps for a zero-point comparison in session 14, using as an example Jenna's belief that she was a "terrible wife" following a small argument with her husband. The therapist asked Jenna to consider what characteristics and behaviors define someone who is a complete failure as a wife, which represents 0% on the continuum (see Figure 5.8). Jenna recognized that a truly "terrible wife" is unfaithful, disrespectful, unhelpful, unloving, unsupportive, verbally abusive, physically abusive,

Quality being rated: _Value as a Wife_

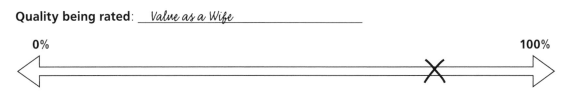

Am I above 0%? How far? (Mark the spot above.)

Define 0%	For what qualities or successes can I give myself credit?
Terrible wife = unfaithful disrespectful unloving unsupportive abusive controlling nagging unwilling to compromise	I support my husband's hobbies & interests I give him backrubs when he is stressed I cook healthy meals for him I contribute to our family income I call his mother regularly We laugh together We help one another with cleaning and errands I love him and am affectionate I plan fun activities for us to do together on the weekends

FIGURE 5.8. Completed Zero-Point Comparisons: Learn to Stop Your Upward Comparisons for Jenna.

and uncompromising. As she completed this exercise, Jenna was able to see that, although imperfect, she was far from a terrible wife. By taking this alternative perspective, she was able to give herself credit for all the times she helped, supported, loved, and cared for her husband. Jenna then practiced zero-point comparisons with other characteristics throughout the next week.

SESSIONS 15–16

The next two treatment sessions focused on body image interventions to help Jenna feel more comfortable and less self-critical at her current weight. This was important for her long-term progress

> *Identify body-checking and avoidance behaviors*

to prevent a return to restrictive dieting and relapse. The therapist reviewed Jenna's responses on the Body Image Checklist (Form B.4 in Appendix B), which she completed as homework between sessions 14 and 15. The Body Image Checklist was used to identify any current checking and avoidance behaviors. Jenna reported that she frequently avoided clothing that showed her shape, frequently checked herself in mirrors, frequently pinched her fat, and sometimes measured

> *Progressive discontinuation of body checking*

parts of her body. Jenna and her therapist reviewed the cognitive-behavioral model of BN, noting how the identified body-checking and body avoidance behaviors both contributed to a distorted view of her body, added to her negative self-image, led to an overemphasis on shape and weight, and left her susceptible to restriction and dieting. Jenna also recognized that she did not feel better or more confident after she engaged in those checking behaviors, and she typically imagined the worst when she engaged in avoidance. As homework, the therapist asked Jenna to discontinue pinching herself over the coming week, and they discussed strategies to resist any urges to do so. After Jenna made it through 1 week without pinching to check her body, she recognized that it was doable. The therapist then requested that Jenna experiment with wearing more revealing clothing on the weekends to disrupt that form of body avoidance. After several weeks of reducing her checking and avoidance behaviors, Jenna noted that she was slightly less focused on her body shape and, as a result, slightly more comfortable with her appearance.

To simultaneously improve her body image, the therapist asked Jenna to track her negative shape-related beliefs. In reviewing her list of negative thoughts, they noticed two basic thought patterns: "I have gained weight, everyone notices how terrible I look, and I am fat and flabby" and "I am out of control; I should do something about my weight before it gets any worse." To challenge these thoughts, Jenna and her therapist completed thought records in session, especially noting evidence that did not support these thoughts: A BMI of 21 indicated she

Cognitive restructuring of body image-related thoughts

was at a healthy weight; she had been receiving positive comments from friends and family; her clothing fit better, and others commented that it looks better on her frame; her energy levels increased; her weight stayed steady within 1 or 2 pounds for the past 5 weeks; and she received more compliments on her appearance from coworkers and strangers. Jenna quickly recognized that her thoughts could still deceive her, that *feeling* fat at any given moment was not the same as *being* fat, that friends she viewed as thin and attractive often said they feel fat, and that being at a higher weight allowed her to be binge- and purge-free. Jenna began a daily practice of noticing positive aspects of her appearance, and she made sure these were not limited to weight-related statements.

The therapist asked Jenna to describe her image of the "perfect" body, and they then together identified the likely costs and benefits if she were able to attain this ideal (see Figure 5.9). Jenna's body ideal was

Identify costs of the "perfect" body

based on a particular supermodel, and the therapist helped her see that this body type represents less than 1% of the population. For most people, including Jenna, to attain this ideal body, one would have to make it a full-time "job," engage in extreme behaviors, and risk multiple health problems. Jenna further recognized that for her to match this ideal, she would have to give up many other important aspects of her life. Even if she did so, this "perfect" body was probably unattainable and thus she would never be happy anyway. To further solidify the advantages of being at her current weight and not devoting her mental energy to maintaining an eating disorder, Jenna's therapist asked her to complete a pie chart representing the most important aspects of her life (see Figure 5.10). At the beginning of

Pie chart exercise

treatment, Jenna's self-image and mental energy were nearly 100% dependent on her body weight. Over the course of treatment to date, Jenna had worked on reinvesting in and developing other important aspects of her life, including her relationship with her husband, her performance at work, and knitting. At the same time, she was practicing holding onto more positive, balanced thoughts about her body shape and appearance.

At this point in treatment, the therapist noted that Jenna had made significant progress. Together, Jenna and the therapist reviewed her improvement since treatment began: no binges in

Describe the "Perfect" Body	Costs of Attaining the "Perfect" Body
102 pounds	Unattainable given my natural shape
Size 2	Would require full-time effort
No flab on abs, hips, or thighs	Restriction, purging, and overexercise
No cellulite	Health problems
Stomach is perfectly flat	Unhappiness
Cannot pinch any fat on waist, arms, or legs	Never satisfied anyway
Legs do not touch one another	No time for anything else that is important
Legs do not jiggle while walking	to me
Can see & feel hip bones	
Perfect hourglass shape	
24-inch waist	

FIGURE 5.9. Completed Costs of the "Perfect" Body for Jenna.

more than 5 weeks, discontinuation of all purging behaviors, the ability to eat a more varied diet, decreased BAI scores, increased comfort around former binge foods, less negative and self-critical thinking, and the ability to cope with and distract herself from emotional triggers and binge urges. The therapist explained that the remainder of treatment would focus on helping Jenna feel more comfortable with her current body weight, to continue challenging persistent negative self-views, and to prepare her posttreatment maintenance plan. These remaining treatment sessions would help ensure that she maintained her progress and was less vulnerable to relapse.

In addition to her many other improvements over the course of treatment, Jenna had slowly gained 13 pounds and now, at 123 pounds, was within the normal weight range (BMI = 21). Although she recognized rationally that she was healthier and happier, felt more in control around food, and looked "normal" at this higher body weight, she had lingering negative thoughts and still feared "getting fat."

SESSIONS 17–18

In past sessions, Jenna and her therapist identified and effectively challenged many of her negative automatic thoughts related to her body, eating, relationships, and general feelings of self-worth. To fur-

Identify interpersonal difficulties

ther target specific destructive thought patterns, the therapist utilized some interpersonal interventions with Jenna. Jenna and her therapist had previously identified several interpersonal problems that were associated with her eating disorder: role transition problems following a recent marriage and a new job, social isolation, and tension and dishonesty in her relationship with her husband. Jenna's primary interpersonal trigger for bingeing, purging, and restriction had been engaging in unhealthy comparisons with other people. Although she did not have trouble eating in front of others, Jenna did feel particularly vulnerable when friends and family discussed dieting or made comments about their own bodies. These interpersonal interactions then trig-

How I saw myself at the beginning of treatment. What was most important to me? How did I evaluate myself?

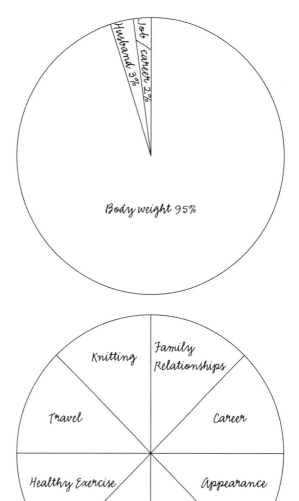

How I would like to see myself. What areas of my life are improved? What else is important to me? Where would I like to invest more time?

FIGURE 5.10. Completed Self-Image Worksheet for Jenna.

gered Jenna to make comparisons between her and others' food intake and appearance. Common thoughts that arose after this type of interaction included: "Everyone is thinner than me"; "Others can eat whatever they want and stay thin"; "If she can diet, I also should be dieting"; "I'm eating more than everyone else at this party so I am a pig." These types of negative automatic thoughts then predictably triggered urges to diet, restrict, or binge, and simultaneously reinforced Jenna's negative perceptions about herself and her body.

During sessions 17 and 18, the therapist helped Jenna monitor and challenge this pattern of unhealthy comparisons with

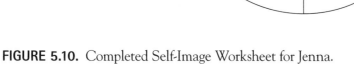

Interpersonal interventions

others. Together, they first identified the cognitive distortions present in these automatic thoughts. In particular, these thoughts were characterized by unfair comparisons, judgment focus, and negative filter. The therapist explained that unfair comparisons were problematic because Jenna focused on the areas in which she felt insecure (e.g., her weight), selectively attended to these qualities in others while not attending to their flaws or insecurities (e.g., financial problems, difficult relationships), and did not factor her own strengths or accomplishments into the comparison (e.g., her husband supported her unconditionally and found her very attractive). Jenna and her therapist then practiced using the seven-column Automatic Thought Records to challenge her unfair comparisons related to weight, appearance, and diet. Jenna's homework was to continue noticing and challenging additional unfair self–other comparisons as they occurred.

Her therapist also used the double-standard technique, in which Jenna was asked to discuss how she defined attractiveness in other people, whether she overemphasized thinness in others, whether she *Additional cognitive restructuring* respected anyone whom she considered unattractive, and whether she knew any thin people whom she considered unattractive. Jenna quickly recognized that her assumption was biased and unfair since she did not hold others to this same standard. In evaluating others' attractiveness, Jenna considered clothing, posture, eyes, skin clarity, smile, hair, projected confidence, and, to a lesser extent, weight. Jenna and her therapist also discussed any historical exceptions to this belief, including that her husband met and fell in love with her when she was at her heaviest adult weight. Jenna's therapist asked her to rewrite her negative thought so that it was more flexible, more attainable, and less punishing. To help, Jenna's therapist asked her to take another perspective on this belief and to consider what advice she might give a friend who held a similar, rigid rule for herself. Jenna revised her thought to be a less perfectionistic rule for herself ("My attractiveness is based on a large number of subjective factors, only one of which is my body weight."), and she was asked to review this revised assumption daily.

As a last interpersonal intervention, the therapist discussed with Jenna how secretive she has been about her eating disorder. Although secrecy is common among patients with eating disorders, Jenna's recovery would be facilitated by having more interpersonal support. Her husband, in particular, was a valuable source of support for her. Although she had not yet been completely honest with him about her eating disorder symptoms, he had the potential to help her through periods of anxiety, intense urges to binge, negative thoughts about herself, and any other potential setback triggers that could arise. Therefore, instead of hiding her eating disorder from her husband out of shame, Jenna agreed to regularly update her husband on her progress, be honest with him if she was having a difficult time, and ask him to help her through particularly difficult situations.

SESSIONS 19–20

In the final two treatment sessions, Jenna and her therapist reviewed the techniques she learned to prevent bingeing, to improve her eating hab- *Relapse prevention* its, and to cope with cravings. The therapist requested that Jenna keep a list of all the useful strategies she learned so that she could reference this list if she had a slip or anticipated a difficult period arising in the future. The therapist also encouraged Jenna to use her social network for support to lower her vulnerability for relapse as she ended treatment. "Red flags," or signs that she was resuming old behaviors and thinking patterns, were identified in the 19th session and throughout the following week: an increase in negative thoughts, temptation to diet or cut out certain foods, resumed bingeing, significant weight loss, eating in secret, and excessive exercise. In the final session, Jenna and her therapist created a detailed relapse plan for each of her "red flags" (see Figure 5.11). Her relapse plan included **Relapse Roadmap** responses such as: resume food records, contact her therapist, use her behavioral strategies list, and resume thought records. After 20 sessions of CBT, in which she was actively involved and fully compliant, Jenna successfully completed treatment.

Bumps in the Road (trigger situations and early signs of relapse)	**Detours from Recovery** (risky responses)	**Seatbelts and Airbags** (healthier, safer alternatives)
• An increase in negative thoughts • Temptation to diet or cut out certain foods • Resume bingeing • Significant weight loss • Eating in secret • Excessive exercise	• Self-criticism • Self–other comparisons • Isolating myself • Bingeing to cope • Dieting and cutting out healthy foods • Rigid food rules • Body checking and pinching • Weighing self multiple times daily • Skipping meals	• Resume food records • Resume regular, planned eating • Challenge negative automatic thoughts • Use walks and breaks to ride out urges • Diaphragmatic breathing for stress • Discontinue body-checking • Talk to husband for support • Review pie chart • Use list of alternative activities • Call therapist

FIGURE 5.11. Completed Relapse Roadmap for Jenna.

CHAPTER 6

Treatment within a Managed Care Context

This treatment planner provides a user-friendly guide to the treatment of BN. Many patients presenting for treatment for an eating disorder will wish to use their health insurance to cover a portion of their treatment costs. Most health insurance companies oversee the cost, quality, and necessity of treatments they will cover. Therapists will, therefore, be required to provide the health insurance company with information pertaining to patients' symptoms, diagnoses, functional impairment, and intended treatment prior to being authorized for treatment sessions. This information will be provided through an initial treatment report, from which the managed care company will then determine the number of sessions and the type of treatment approved. The presence and severity of symptoms, combined with the use of a treatment specifically targeting those symptoms, are the primary factors that determine approval by managed care companies.

Because CBT is an empirically supported, effective, short-term treatment, it is particularly well suited for use within a managed care system. There are three basic areas of overlap between CBT and the priorities of managed care organizations. Both CBT and managed care companies (1) define the symptoms themselves as the problem; (2) emphasize symptom relief as the explicit goal of treatment; and (3) consider treatment effective if it reduces these symptoms. As we stressed earlier, BN is a serious psychological disorder that is chronic without treatment. Thus, health insurance companies recognize the need for treatment for eating disorders. In particular, the empirically supported CBT protocol for BN provided in this book is highly compatible with the aims of managed care companies.

This chapter provides therapists with guidelines to work efficiently and effectively with health care insurance reviewers, where the common goal is to ensure that patients receive coverage for an adequate course of treatment sessions. Information provided in this chapter will guide you through:

- Understanding covered treatments and diagnoses.
- Describing the treatment and intended interventions.
- Progress updates.
- Paperwork, including initial treatment reports and requests for additional sessions.

GETTING APPROVAL FOR TREATMENTS

Managed care companies are committed to controlling costs while simultaneously ensuring that their enrollees receive treatments that are both necessary and effective. Because BN is a recognized psychological disorder with multiple medical, emotional, and functional consequences, patients with BN symptoms usually meet the standards for medical necessity (described next). Therapists using the included treatment protocol should have little trouble obtaining approval for patient sessions, since CBT works efficiently and effectively to reduce symptoms. Proper communication with the managed care companies will still be required, however.

Medical Necessity

Medical necessity is a precondition for treatment approval by most insurance companies. Insurance companies will evaluate whether treatment is medically necessary based on a patient's psychiatric diagnosis, type and severity of symptoms, Global Assessment of Functioning (GAF) score, and degree of functional impairment. Psychiatric diagnosis is generated from the current version of the DSM.* Typically, the eating disorder diagnoses BN (DSM-IV-TR code: 307.51) and AN (DSM-IV-TR code: 307.1) are covered by insurance companies. By definition, BN and AN involve severe symptoms and significant impairment in functioning. EDNOS (DSM-IV-TR code: 307.50) may be covered as well, although the therapist will need to explain the type and severity of symptoms. In DSM-IV-TR, BED, purging disorder, and subthreshold eating disorders fall under the diagnostic category of EDNOS. It should be noted that psychological treatments for obesity (without binge eating) are not typically covered by managed care companies, while treatment for BED can be covered.

The therapist will be required to describe the patient's presenting problem beyond the diagnosis. When describing the patient's eating disorder and comorbid psychological symptoms, the therapist should designate whether the symptoms are mild, moderate, or severe. Functional impairment can include any disruption in the patient's social, occupational, educational, and familial functioning. Medical consequences of the eating disorder also should be detailed because these suggest that treatment is medically necessary. In addition, certain symptoms of BN are especially indicative of the need for immediate treatment: purging, low body weight, and excessive exercise. Severe comorbid symptoms, such as suicidality and a depressed mood, will also contribute to a determination for medical necessity.

Appropriate Treatment

When determining approval for a course of psychological treatment, "appropriate treatment" is the second basic consideration for insurance companies. Treatments are usually deemed appro-

---

*At the time of printing, the current version of the DSM is DSM-IV-TR. An updated version, DSM-5, is expected in 2013. Changes are expected to several diagnostic categories within the eating disorders and to specific symptoms for diagnostic criteria.

priate if they are at a suitable level of care, include interventions targeted to the patient's primary symptoms, are comprehensive, and are known to be efficacious for meeting the patient's treatment goals. The CBT protocol described in this book will be considered appropriate in most instances since its interventions are empirically supported and its primary goals are symptom reduction.

We discussed level-of-care considerations in Chapter 1. In general, an insurance company is unlikely to cover more intensive treatment (e.g., inpatient or twice-weekly sessions) than is warranted given the patient's symptom severity. The therapist may be asked to justify a request for more frequent treatment sessions.

Managed care companies will also want the therapist to demonstrate that treatment is comprehensive, meaning that it is sufficient to treat the eating disorder. At times, concurrent care by a psychiatrist, internist, and/or nutritionist may be required to qualify as appropriate treatment. The therapist may be asked to justify the patient receiving treatment in the absence of care by these other providers.

THE INITIAL TREATMENT REPORT

Managed care companies may require initial treatment plans and/or treatment progress reports before approving your patient's sessions. Most health insurance companies provide their own form for filing treatment reports. Other companies request a written statement from the therapist without recommending any particular structure for the report. In either case, both initial treatment plans and treatment progress reports should include the following information: the patient's primary and secondary diagnoses, presenting problem, mental status examination results, and treatment plan. Each of these areas is described in more detail next. A sample initial treatment report and a sample request for additional outpatient treatment sessions for the case of Jenna are provided in Figures 6.1 and 6.2, respectively.

Diagnosis

The therapist will provide the managed care company with complete diagnostic information. Complete information about the multiaxial classification system, diagnostic categories, and diagnostic codes, including the five diagnostic axes, can be found in the DSM. The current version is the DSM-IV-TR (American Psychiatric Association, 2000). The five diagnostic axes require the therapist to describe the patient's immediate, primary disorders (Axis I); any personality disorder, developmental disorder, learning disability, or mental retardation (Axis II); medical or neurological problems (Axis III); significant psychosocial stressors (Axis IV); and level of functioning (Axis V). Care should be taken to ensure accurate diagnosis, including all primary and comorbid conditions for which the patient meets diagnostic criteria. Underdiagnosing a patient may result in approval for too little treatment, while overdiagnosing a patient is unethical. The therapist will rely on the patient's report, clinical assessment, self-report measures, and DSM diagnostic criteria to determine diagnoses.

Symptoms

Diagnosis

Axis I	Bulimia nervosa (307.51)	
	Generalized anxiety disorder (300.02)	
Axis II	Obsessive–compulsive personality disorder (301.4)	
Axis III	Slightly underweight; No other conditions or allergies reported	
Axis IV	Stressors related to employment, recent marriage, family, recent move, and reduced social support network	
Axis V	Current: GAF = 55	
	Highest past year: GAF = 55	

Presenting Problem

Jenna Smith is a 26-year-old female with an extended history of bulimia nervosa. She has been bingeing and purging for the 6 years prior to treatment intake. Currently, she reports bingeing and purging approximately twice daily. She sought treatment at this time because of concerns about the severity of her eating disorder and because it is affecting her health, work performance, and intimate relationship. She has had no prior psychological or psychiatric treatment.

Symptoms

Bingeing twice daily	Poor body image
Purging twice daily	Overevaluation of own shape/weight
Dietary restriction	Borderline underweight (BMI = 19)
Rigid dietary rules	Intense fear of weight gain
Poor concentration	Anxiety (BAI = 27)
Chronic worry	

Strengths

High motivation for change	Good insight
Stable employment	High intelligence
Supportive intimate relationship	Stable mood

Functioning

Because of the severity and chronicity of her eating disorder and anxiety symptoms, this patient is experiencing mild to moderate impairment in her work, intimate relationship, and social functioning. She has no current or past suicidal or homicidal ideation.

Mental Status

At intake, this patient was fully oriented, was well groomed, and displayed appropriate behavior, affect, speech, and thought processes. She denied current or past hallucinations. She exhibited good insight and judgment, and she was fully cooperative with this therapist.

Goals and Interventions

Treatment Goals

Eliminate bingeing	Decrease anxiety symptoms
Eliminate purging	Increase body weight to healthy range
Reduce dietary restriction	Improve body image
Improve urge coping skills	Improve work performance/concentration

(cont.)

FIGURE 6.1. Sample Initial Treatment Report for Jenna.

Planned Interventions

Bibliotherapy and psychoeducation for eating disorder and anxiety
Behavioral alternatives to bingeing
Daily food records
Weekly weighing
Problem-solving skills
Cognitive restructuring
Relaxation training
Urge coping skills
Reintroduce restricted foods
Body image interventions
Relapse prevention
Referral to psychiatrist for medication consultation

Medication

Patient is not currently on any psychotropic medications. A referral will be provided to a psychiatrist for a consultation to address her anxiety symptoms and bingeing.

Expected Treatment

Modality: Individual sessions
Frequency: Once weekly
Duration: 20 weeks

FIGURE 6.1 (*cont.*)

Axis I

Axis I diagnoses cover all childhood and adult clinical disorders and life areas requiring clinical attention (e.g., V codes) except the personality disorders and mental retardation, which are recorded on Axis II. All relevant psychological disorders, including any comorbid conditions, should be included on the treatment report. This is important for relaying severity of the presenting problem and potential complications with treatment.

When communicating with insurance companies, the therapist may be asked to differentiate the principal diagnosis from secondary diagnoses. In an outpatient setting, the principal diagnosis is the patient's stated reason for the visit. When obtaining authorization to treat an eating disorder, this diagnosis (e.g., BN) should be listed as the principal diagnosis. Be sure to include subtype specifiers, where appropriate (e.g., AN, nonpurging type). Secondary diagnoses include any other disorder for which the patient meets full criteria. The principal diagnosis should be listed first on the treatment report.

Axis II

When applicable, all personality disorder diagnoses and mental retardation should be listed on Axis II. The patient may meet criteria for a single Axis II diagnosis or a cluster of diagnoses. Although not the central focus of eating disorder treatment, personality disorders and/or mental

Patient Information

Name: _____ *Jenna Smith* _____
Patient ID #: _____ - _____ - _____

Provider Information

Name: _____
License Number: _____

ICD-9 / DSM-IV Diagnosis

Axis I: *307.51 (primary)* _____
            300.02 (secondary) _____
Axis II: *301.4* _____
Axis III: *No conditions or allergies reported* _____
Axis IV: *Stressors related to employment, marriage,* _____
            family, recent move, and social _____
Axis V: *Current: GAF = 60* _____
            At intake: GAF = 55 _____

Functional Impairment

(check if applicable)	Mild	Moderate	Severe
Activities of daily living	❑	❑	❑
Relationships	☑	❑	❑
Work/school	☑	❑	❑
Physical health	☑	❑	❑

Treatment began on: _08_ / _17_ / _08_

___6___ # sessions to date

Improvement to Date: ❑ None   ❑ Minor   ☑ Moderate   ❑ Significant

Current Symptom Severity

(check if applicable)	Mild	Moderate	Severe
Anxiety	❑	☑	❑
Decreased energy	☑	❑	❑
Delusions	❑	❑	❑
Depressed mood	❑	❑	❑
Hallucinations	❑	❑	❑
Hopelessness	❑	❑	❑
Hyperactivity	❑	❑	❑
Inattention	☑	❑	❑
Irritability	☑	❑	❑
Panic attacks	❑	❑	❑
Sleep disturbance	❑	❑	❑

(cont.)

FIGURE 6.2. Sample Request for Additional Outpatient Treatment Sessions for Jenna.

Treatment Goals

#1 _Remain binge/purge-free while stabilizing at a healthy weight_
#2 _Improve body image_

Risk Evaluation

Suicidal: ☐ Ideation   ☐ Plan   ☐ Intent   ☐ Prior attempt
Homicidal: ☐ Ideation   ☐ Plan   ☐ Intent   ☐ Prior attempt
Self-injurious behavior: ☐ Current   ☐ Past

Requested # Additional Sessions: _____12_____

FIGURE 6.2 (*cont.*)

retardation will complicate the expected course and duration of treatment. Stated treatment goals, however, should still target resolution of the eating disorder symptoms. When no Axis II condition is met, the code V71.09 should be used. To defer diagnosis on Axis II, use code 799.99.

Axis III

The therapist should list all current medical conditions and known allergies on Axis III. This includes medical conditions associated with the eating disorder (e.g., obesity, low body weight, low blood pressure) as well as unrelated conditions (e.g., diabetes).

Axis IV

All current psychosocial stressors should be reported on Axis IV. These may include (but are not limited to) stressors related to social support, intimate relationships, role changes, education, occupation, housing, finances, access to health care, legal, or trauma history. Some stressors result from the eating disorder and others arise independently. Because any significant stressor may maintain the eating disorder or complicate treatment, the therapist should clearly note all stressors on the treatment reports.

Axis V

The therapist will provide a summary score of the patient's level of functioning, or GAF score. A detailed description of GAF scores can be found in the DSM-IV-TR (American Psychiatric Association, 2000). GAF scores are determined by the therapist and are based on the severity of psychological symptoms and the degree of functional impairment. GAF scores range from 0–100, with lower GAF scores indicating more severe impairment. It is customary to note the patient's GAF score at intake as well as the highest level of functioning in the past year (see Figure 6.1).

Managed care representatives will use the GAF score to help determine the appropriate level of care and expected duration of treatment for patients. A GAF score below 30 or 40 may suggest the need for inpatient treatment, 35–69 suggests outpatient treatment is warranted, and above 65 or 70 suggests mental health treatment is not needed, except in the case of managing a chronic, serious condition (New Avenues, 2003).

Presenting Problem

In the next section of the initial treatment report, the therapist provides additional information about the patient's psychological problem beyond diagnoses.

Eating Disorder Symptoms

Any clinically significant symptoms that will be addressed in treatment should be listed here. It is important for the therapist to include all eating disorder symptoms the patient exhibits, because the managed care reviewer will want to confirm that the patient meets diagnostic criteria. Symptoms should be listed just as they appear in the current DSM. You may also wish to consult Table 6.1 for a listing of common symptoms of BN.

Comorbid Symptoms

Comorbid psychological symptoms should also be included in the initial treatment report, particularly those that will impact the course of treatment or those that will be addressed concurrently with the eating disorder. Because most patients with BN meet criteria for another Axis I disorder, symptoms of depression, obsessive–compulsive disorder, social anxiety, or substance abuse may be present.

Strengths

Some initial treatment reports ask for the patient's strengths in addition to psychological symptoms. Strengths are personal or environmental characteristics that may contribute to a positive

TABLE 6.1. Sample Symptoms of Bulimia Nervosa

• Binge episodes (indicate frequency)	• Lack of enjoyment in usual activities
• Purging: vomiting, laxative use, enemas, diuretics (specify type and frequency)	• Social anxiety
• Dietary restriction	• Irritability
• Rigid dietary rules	• Depressed mood
• Excessive exercise	• Low motivation
• Low body weight	• Self-criticism
• Overweight/obesity	• Excessive shame and guilt
• Poor body image	• Feelings of worthlessness
• Overevaluation of shape/weight	• Suicidal ideation
• Social avoidance	• Poor distress tolerance

treatment outcome. The therapist may wish to include intelligence, strong motivation, stable employment, supportive relationships, or a positive response to past treatments.

Functional Impairment

Specific ways in which the patient's symptoms interfere with optimal functioning should be described. Many patients with an eating disorder will experience disruptions in their ability to work, attend school, socialize, maintain an intimate relationship, meet familial obligations, and parent.

Threat to Self or Others

If the patient reports any current or past suicidality, homicidality, or self-injurious behavior, this should be clearly noted on the initial treatment report since these impact treatment necessity. For any suicidality or homicidality, clearly denote whether the patient reports ideation, plan, intent, access to means, or a past attempt.

Mental Status Examination

The Mental Status Examination is one part of clinical assessment that provides descriptive information about a patient's observable presentation. The therapist should assess the patient at intake and provide mental status information in the initial treatment report. Many insurance companies will provide a mental status checklist on their treatment request forms. If no form is provided, the therapist will instead provide a brief written description using the mental status categories (and their respective descriptors) outlined next:

- **Appearance:** well groomed, disheveled, bizarre, or inappropriate
- **Attitude:** cooperative, uncooperative, hostile, guarded, suspicious, or regressed
- **Orientation:** fully oriented or impaired orientation to person, place, time, or purpose
- **Motor activity:** calm, hyperactive, agitated, tremors, tics, or muscle spasms
- **Attention:** good, fair, easily distracted, or highly distractible
- **Mood:** normal, depressed, anxious, or elevated
- **Affect:** appropriate, labile, expansive, constricted, or blunted
- **Speech:** normal, slow, slurred, pressured, or rapid
- **Thought process:** intact, circumstantial, tangential, flight of ideas, or loose associations
- **Hallucinations:** none, auditory, visual, olfactory, or command
- **Delusions:** none, persecutory, grandiose, or religious
- **Memory:** intact or impairment in immediate, short-term, or long-term memory
- **Insight:** able or not able to recognize symptoms as mental illness

Treatment

The therapist will need to propose a course and expected length of treatment on the initial treatment report. Managed care companies are particularly concerned with whether proposed treatments will target and effectively resolve the patient's psychological symptoms. Thus, the initial treatment report will include a list of **specific treatment goals** as well as **interventions** to be used to meet those goals. See Table 6.2 for sample treatment goals and interventions for BN, which will be useful in writing this section of the report. Treatment goals should be both observable and measurable, whenever possible. Goals may include elimination of specific symptoms, behavioral change, increased functioning in specific life areas, weight gain or loss, improved body image, or cognitive change. Proposed treatment interventions should directly target the outlined goals. The cognitive-behavioral interventions described in this book can be listed for this section of the initial treatment report. See the 20-session sample treatment plan in Chapter 4 for a comprehensive listing of BN interventions. Concise descriptions of the proposed **modality of treatment** (e.g., individual or group therapy), expected **frequency of sessions,** expected **duration of treatment,** and any concurrent psychotropic **medication** should also be listed.

A sample initial treatment report is provided in Figure 6.1 to further assist therapists in their reports to managed care companies. The sample report is based on the case example from Chapter 5, including this patient's presenting problem, symptoms at intake, diagnoses, assessment results, and level of impairment. Treatment goals, interventions, and expected frequency/

TABLE 6.2. Sample Treatment Goals and Interventions for Bulimia Nervosa

Treatment goals	Interventions
• Eliminate bingeing	• Bibliotherapy, food records, stimulus control, alternative behaviors, problem solving
• Eliminate purging	• Psychoeducation, delay, test negative predictions, relaxation training, alternative behaviors
• Improve urge coping skills	• Relaxation training, urge surfing
• Reduce dietary restriction	• Cognitive restructuring, reintroduce restricted foods, test negative predictions
• Increase body weight to BMI > 20	• Psychoeducation, weekly weighing, regular eating, reintroduce restricted foods
• Improve mood	• Activity schedule, cognitive restructuring
• Increase social participation	• Problem solving, activity schedule
• Reduce negative automatic thoughts	• Identify cognitive distortions, cognitive restructuring
• Modify perfectionistic beliefs	• Cognitive restructuring, behavioral experiments, double-standard technique
• Improve body image	• Cognitive restructuring, pie chart exercise, reduce checking/avoidance behaviors, positive data log
• Develop relapse coping skills	• Identify "red-flag" signs, review effective techniques, relapse coping card

duration are based on the treatment plans provided in this book, and these will apply to most patients presenting for treatment for BN.

In some instances, a managed care representative reviews the proposed treatment by speaking with the therapist by phone. The therapist can effectively prepare for the call by outlining the patient's diagnostic and symptom information. Regardless of the format in which case information is presented to the insurance company, the therapist should obtain a release of information from the patient and should safeguard the patient's confidentiality and protected health information. Further, the importance of accurately reporting a patient's diagnosis and treatment plans cannot be overstated. The therapist is both legally and ethically obligated to accurately convey the patient's intended treatment, diagnosis, symptoms, and functional impairment.

REQUESTS FOR ADDITIONAL SESSIONS

Although the expected course of CBT for BN is 20 sessions, managed care companies typically approve no more than 10 sessions at the outset of treatment. Initial coverage is provided with the understanding that additional sessions can be requested later. Often the therapist will be asked to complete a request form specific to the insurance company, although occasionally requests are reviewed by telephone. The therapist will be asked to justify continued treatment by demonstrating that the patient had an early response to treatment but still exhibits significant psychological symptoms and impaired functioning. Managed care companies are unlikely to approve additional treatment sessions if there has been no improvement as they will want to ensure efficacious care. Likewise, if the patient has made substantial progress and no longer exhibits significant psychological symptoms, then there is no demonstrable need for additional treatment sessions. If the patient has made less progress than expected as a result of new symptoms or environmental factors since the initial treatment report, or if any new diagnostic information has arisen, this should be clearly reported on requests for additional treatment sessions.

Requests for additional treatment often include many of the same elements as an initial treatment report, including diagnoses, current symptoms, degree of impairment, mental status, risk evaluation, treatment goals, and planned treatment interventions (see Figure 6.2). The therapist should reference the initial treatment report and provide an update for all the areas just outlined. For example, progress to date should be reported for each of the original treatment goals written in the initial treatment report. The therapist should note whether the patient has made substantial, moderate, some, or no progress toward each of the original goals.

The therapist will also need to address whether there are any changes or improvement in the patient's diagnoses, symptom presentation, functional impairment, and mental status. All current symptoms and functional impairment will be recorded, including both symptoms originally described at intake and any new symptoms.

There will be space for the therapist to record current treatment goals, which may be similar to or revised since intake. Any new or continuing treatment goals should also be listed in all requests for additional treatment. Treatment goals will be based on the patient's early response to treatment and any new information brought to the therapist's attention. It should be noted that relapse prevention is a worthy treatment goal. The therapist will likely need to outline intended interventions for the remaining sessions, and these should match the updated treatment goals.

Finally, the therapist will need to request a set number of sessions for the continuation of treatment. The number of requested sessions should be based on what remains of the recommended 20-session treatment protocol, with adjustments made for rapid progress, setbacks, or significant comorbidity. Justification for the number of requested sessions should be apparent based on the treatment goals and progress to date already reported by the therapist elsewhere on the request form.

Additional treatment sessions are more likely to be permitted and covered if the patient exhibits any combination of the following:

1. Suicidality or homicidality
2. Severe and persistent symptoms
3. Impairment in daily living, physical, familial, social, occupational, educational, and/or relationship functioning
4. Concurrent affective disorder, alcohol abuse, or substance abuse
5. A life crisis that arose since the last treatment report
6. Evidence of improvement in symptoms since the last treatment report

It is worth reemphasizing that CBT for BN is highly compatible with working within the managed care system because it is focused on a direct, rapid reduction in psychological symptoms. Although communicating with insurance companies can be intimidating or difficult at times, the therapist should always strive for accuracy in reporting symptoms, progress, and diagnoses, as ethical practice is always in the patient's best interest.

APPENDIX A

"Transdiagnosis" of Eating Disorders

Because AN, BN, and EDNOS are part of an imperfect categorical diagnostic system, and all eating disorders share similar core symptoms, several experts now suggest a "transdiagnostic" approach to the assessment and treatment of eating disorders (Fairburn et al., 2003). Rather than labeling BN, BED, and other variations of EDNOS as distinct disorders requiring unique treatments, Fairburn and colleagues suggest that the eating disorders share several common maintaining mechanisms and thus will respond to a unified treatment protocol.

There is a strong symptomatic overlap among the eating disorders, as described in Chapter 1. There is also overlap across time, since many individuals progress from one eating disorder to another in their lifetime (often AN into BN or BN into a chronic form of EDNOS; Tozzi et al., 2005). Not only do the eating disorders share many common symptoms, cognitions, and behavioral patterns, but the diagnostic categories themselves have been shown to be imperfect. Research suggests that EDNOS does not serve as a residual category, as intended, but is instead the most common diagnosis among patients with eating disorders. Lifetime prevalence for EDNOS is estimated to be 2.4%, which is more than three times the combined lifetime prevalence for AN and BN (Machado et al., 2007). EDNOS accounts for approximately half of all inpatient and outpatient eating disorder treatment sessions (Button et al., 2005). Just as with AN and BN, significant proportions of patients with an EDNOS diagnosis restrict their daily food intake, overexercise, vomit, abuse laxatives, have comorbid depression, experience suicidal ideation, have intense fears of weight gain, and report body image disturbances (Button et al., 2005; Wade, 2007).

Fairburn and colleagues (2009) developed a "transdiagnostic" cognitive-behavioral treatment program that targets the core eating disorder symptoms and can be utilized in most outpatient eating disorder cases. In testing this approach, the transdiagnostic treatment was found to work well for nearly all patients regardless of initial diagnosis (provided initial body weight was not in the underweight range) (Fairburn et al., 2009; Helverskov et al., 2010). This research suggests that outpatient treatment for eating disorders should not be diagnostically driven but should instead target the common eating disorder symptoms, an individual's core symptoms, and any unique presenting complications.

EDNOS is a diagnosis met by patients with clinically significant and often medically dangerous eating disorders, including BED and purging disorder (Button et al., 2005; Fairburn et al., 2007). BED is currently diagnosed in the EDNOS catch-all category. Although EDNOS also serves as the diagnosis for individuals with subthreshold eating disorders, these eating disorders may be just as significant as AN and BN. For example, individuals who meet all diagnostic criteria for AN except amenorrhea have severe eating disorders nearly indistinguishable from those of their counterparts meeting full diagnostic criteria (Roberto, Steinglass, Mayer, Attia, & Walsh, 2008). Individuals with subthreshold AN or BN typically have just as many prior hospitalizations, comorbid depression and anxiety, and illnesses of similar duration as those with AN or BN, although they do have a higher BMI (Fairburn et al., 2007; Roberto et al., 2008). The early research on EDNOS suggests that individuals with clinically significant eating disorders, even if they do not meet diagnostic criteria for BN or AN, warrant targeted and effective psychological treatments that are similar to the well-researched, empirically supported treatments for BN.

Therefore, although accurate diagnosis is an important first step in the assessment of eating disorders, it is important to recognize the significant overlap among them. All effective treatments should target both the common core features of the eating disorders as well as a patient's idiosyncratic symptom presentation. The cognitive-behavioral treatment plan for BN presented in this book can be readily adapted to patients with eating disorders with overlapping symptom presentations, particularly those with subthreshold BN, purging disorder, and BED.

Selected Assessment Tools

APPENDIX B.1. EVALUATION OF EATING DISORDERS

The Evaluation of Eating Disorders is a semistructured clinical interview intended for use in the first session with a patient. This evaluation includes all relevant areas for assessing the patient's current and past eating disorder symptom severity, mental status, comorbid symptoms, medical health, suicidality, food intake, cognitions, relationships, emotional triggers, personal strengths, and treatment goals. The Evaluation of Eating Disorders provides structure for the assessment phase of treatment. The therapist can administer the Evaluation of Eating Disorders by asking the patient each of the questions and recording the patient's responses on the form.

The Evaluation of Eating Disorders will guide the therapist in making level-of-care decisions, case conceptualization, and selection of treatment interventions. As outlined in Chapter 1, the patient who reports severe eating disorder symptoms (e.g., severely underweight), medical complications, repeated failed outpatient episodes, or significant suicidality may require immediate referral to a higher level of care. For the patient for whom outpatient treatment is deemed appropriate, the Evaluation of Eating Disorders provides the therapist with extensive information for case conceptualization and treatment planning. The eating disorder symptoms, specific cognitions, comorbid depression and anxiety, interpersonal problems, and emotional triggers endorsed by the patient should be included in the case conceptualization (see Form 3.2). As treatment begins, the therapist will tailor treatment interventions to ensure that the patient's behavioral, cognitive, interpersonal, and emotional problems are adequately addressed, while unnecessary treatment interventions need not be included in the treatment plan. For example, a patient with BED who does not purge will not require interventions for compensatory behaviors, and a patient with a positive, supportive social network will not require interpersonal interventions. Likewise, a patient with notable dietary restriction and a low body weight will benefit from particular focus throughout treatment on regular eating, reincorporating restricted foods, and cognitive restructuring interventions.

FORM B.1.   Evaluation of Eating Disorders

Patient's name: _____   Date: _____

MENTAL STATE

Notes on patient's mental state, orientation, presentation, speech, and interpersonal demeanor:

_____

_____

_____

CURRENT SYMPTOMS

Presenting problem ("Why are you seeking treatment now?"): _____

_____

Current weight: _____

Height: _____

Body mass index: _____

Date of last menstrual period: _____

Use of hormonal birth control: _____

Frequency of bingeing: _____

Vomiting frequency: _____

Laxative use: _____

Last physical exam (date and results): _____

_____

Current medications (including doses): _____

_____

Eating Disorders Examination Questionnaire (EDE-Q) scores: _____

   Restraint subscale: _____

   Eating Concern subscale: _____

   Shape Concern subscale: _____

   Weight Concern subscale: _____

Clinical Impairment Assessment Questionnaire (CIA) score: _____

(cont.)

SYMPTOM HISTORY

Lowest adult weight (date): _____

Highest adult weight (date): _____

Date of onset of bulimia symptoms: _____

Any periods of remission: _____

Prior treatment (dates and outcome): _____

_____

_____

Past hospitalizations: _____

_____

_____

Past medications: _____

_____

_____

COMORBID SYMPTOMS

Beck Depression Inventory (BDI) score: _____
    (0–13 = minimal depression; 14–19 = mild depression; 20–28 = moderate depression; 29–63 = severe
    depression [Beck, Steer, & Brown, 1996])

Beck Anxiety Inventory (BAI) score: _____
    (0–7 = minimal anxiety; 8–15 = mild anxiety; 16–25 = moderate anxiety; 26–63 = severe anxiety [Beck &
    Steer, 1993])

"Have you ever been in treatment for other psychological concerns?" _____

_____

Depressive symptoms (current or past): _____

Anxiety symptoms (current or past): _____

_____

Alcohol and substance use (current or past; frequency and quantity; any consequences of use; concern about
own use): _____

Personality traits: _____

_____

_____

Suicidal ideation or fantasies about death: _____

If yes, see Form B.8 (Evaluation of Suicide Risk)

Prior suicide attempts (dates, method, severity): _____

_____

_____

(cont.)

BEHAVIORS

"Describe a typical day's food intake": _____

_____

_____

"Do you skip meals and/or intentionally diet?" _____

"Describe a typical binge." _____

_____

_____

Common binge triggers: _____

_____

_____

Body Image Checklist scores: _____

    Avoidance subscale: _____

    Checking subscale: _____

    Dissatisfaction subscale: _____

COGNITIONS

Elicit patient's thoughts about body shape, current weight, safe foods, restricted foods, and food rules (e.g., "I am fat and my thighs are gross"; "I should be a size 2"; "I can't eat sugar without losing control"): _____

_____

_____

Eating Disorder Belief Questionnaire (EDBQ) scores: _____

    Negative Self-Beliefs subscale: _____

    Acceptance by Others subscale: _____

    Self-Acceptance subscale: _____

    Control over Eating subscale: _____

RELATIONSHIPS

Family members: _____

_____

Relationship with family: _____

_____

Intimate relationship status (duration; prior notable relationships): _____

_____

"Do your family and friends know about your eating disorder?" _____

_____

(cont.)

"How supportive is your family of you seeking treatment?" _____

_____

"Do you eat/binge/purge in secret?" _____

"Do you feel pressure from family, friends, coworkers, or society to be thin?" _____

_____

Familial history of eating disorders, depression, anxiety, and substance abuse: _____

_____

EMOTIONS

"Describe how you feel before and after a binge": _____

_____

_____

"Describe how you feel before and after purging": _____

_____

_____

"How do you handle intense emotions? What do you do?" _____

_____

_____

"How long do these intense emotions last?" _____

STRENGTHS

Patient's self-described and apparent strengths (e.g., intelligent, insightful, educated, good social support network, strong family support, highly motivated, good coping skills): _____

_____

_____

INITIAL TREATMENT GOALS

"What do you hope to get out of this treatment?" "What are your goals in terms of symptoms, mood, and thinking?" _____

_____

_____

"How motivated do you feel for treatment?" (on a scale of 1–10; describe) _____

_____

"What might get in the way of you succeeding in treatment?" _____

_____

APPENDIX B.2. EATING DISORDERS
EXAMINATION QUESTIONNAIRE (EDE-Q)

The Eating Disorders Examination Questionnaire (EDE-Q) is a self-report measure that can be used to assess the presence and frequency of many eating disorder behaviors over the preceding 28 days. The EDE-Q assesses bingeing, purging, dietary restriction, body image, and fear of weight gain. It provides the therapist with information about the relative severity of eating concerns, body shape concerns, and weight concerns, which make up the measure's three subscales. It is appropriate for use with patients with a range of disordered eating, including those with AN, BN, and EDNOS. The EDE-Q has demonstrated reliability and validity, and normative scores are provided with the scoring instructions. Therefore, it can be used for both clinical and research purposes. The EDE-Q, its scoring information, and community norms are provided here with permission from its developers.

Because the EDE-Q is a self-report measure, the therapist should ask the patient to complete the assessment on her own before intake or between sessions. Instructions for the patient are provided on the EDE-Q. Typically, the therapist will use the EDE-Q to assess eating disorder symptoms and severity at intake and again at the end of treatment.

After the patient has completed the EDE-Q, the therapist will score the responses. Global and subscale scores are calculated as the mean score on the relevant questions. The resulting score ranges from 0 to 6, with a higher score indicating more severe eating disorder pathology in that area. The included community norms provide additional context for the severity of the patient's eating disorder. For example, a patient's global EDE-Q score of 2.9 is more than 1 standard deviation above the community norm and, therefore, indicates an eating disorder that warrants clinical attention. A global or subscale score in the normative range does not rule out the presence of an eating disorder and does not preclude a patient from having symptoms that are distressing or interfere with functioning. Patients often have elevated scores on only select subscales (e.g., Eating Concern, Weight Concern, and Shape Concern but not Restraint), and this provides the therapist with additional information about which areas require the most clinical intervention. In this way, the patient's individual responses, total score, and subscale scores can then assist the therapist with case conceptualization and treatment planning. The therapist can also utilize EDE-Q responses and scores to provide the patient with feedback about the severity of her eating disorder.

EDE-Q SCORING INFORMATION

Introduction

The EDE-Q is a self-report version of the Eating Disorder Examination (EDE), the well-established investigator-based interview (Fairburn & Cooper, 1993). It is scored in the same way as the EDE. Its performance has been compared with that of the EDE: In some respects it performs well, but in others it does not.

Source: Fairburn and Beglin (2008).

Scoring

The EDE-Q generates two types of data. First, it provides frequency data on key behavioral features of eating disorders in terms of number of episodes of the behavior and in some instances number of days on which the behavior has occurred. Second, it provides subscale scores reflecting the severity of aspects of the psychopathology of eating disorders. The subscales are Restraint, Eating Concern, Shape Concern, and Weight Concern. To obtain a particular subscale score, the ratings for the relevant items (listed below) are added together and the sum is divided by the total number of items forming the subscale. If ratings are only available on some items, a score may nevertheless be obtained by dividing the resulting total by the number of rated items so long as more than half the items have been rated. To obtain an overall or "global" score, the four subscales are summed and the resulting total divided by the number of subscales (i.e., four).

Subscale Items

Restraint

1 Restraint over eating
2 Avoidance of eating
3 Food avoidance
4 Dietary rules
5 Empty stomach

Eating Concern

7   Preoccupation with food, eating, or calories
9   Fear of losing control over eating
19 Eating in secret
21 Social eating
20 Guilt about eating

Shape Concern

6   Flat stomach
8   Preoccupation with shape or weight
23 Importance of shape
10 Fear of weight gain
26 Dissatisfaction with shape
27 Discomfort seeing body
28 Avoidance of exposure
11 Feelings of fatness

Weight Concern

22 Importance of weight
24 Reaction to prescribed weight
8   Preoccupation with shape or weight
25 Dissatisfaction with weight
12 Desire to lose weight

Community Norms

The data below are from a community-based sample of young women (N = 241) assessed using the EDE-Q.

Global EDE-Q (four subscales)	1.554 (± 1.213)
Restraint subscale	1.251 (± 1.323)
Eating Concern subscale	0.624 (± 0.859)
Shape Concern subscale	2.149 (± 1.602)
Weight Concern subscale	1.587 (± 1.369)

FORM B.2. Eating Disorders Examination Questionnaire (EDE-Q)

VERSION 6.0   Copyright 2008 by Christopher Fairburn and Sarah Beglin

Instructions: The following questions are concerned with the past 4 weeks (28 days) only. Please read each question carefully. Please answer all the questions. Thank you.

Questions 1–12: Please circle the appropriate number on the right. Remember that the questions refer to the past 4 weeks (28 days) only.

On how many of the past 28 days ...	No days	1–5 days	6–12 days	13–15 days	16–22 days	23–27 days	Every day
1. Have you been deliberately *trying* to limit the amount of food you eat to influence your shape or weight (whether or not you have succeeded)?	0	1	2	3	4	5	6
2. Have you gone for long periods of time (8 waking hours or more) without eating anything at all in order to influence your shape or weight?	0	1	2	3	4	5	6
3. Have you *tried* to exclude from your diet any foods that you like in order to influence your shape or weight (whether or not you have succeeded)?	0	1	2	3	4	5	6
4. Have you *tried* to follow definite rules regarding your eating (for example, a calorie limit) in order to influence your shape or weight (whether or not you have succeeded)?	0	1	2	3	4	5	6
5. Have you had a definite desire to have an *empty* stomach with the aim of influencing your shape or weight?	0	1	2	3	4	5	6
6. Have you had a definite desire to have a *totally flat* stomach?	0	1	2	3	4	5	6
7. Has thinking about *food, eating or calories* made it very difficult to concentrate on things you are interested in (for example, working, following a conversation, or reading)?	0	1	2	3	4	5	6
8. Has thinking about *shape or weight* made it very difficult to concentrate on things you are interested in (for example, working, following a conversation, or reading)?	0	1	2	3	4	5	6

(cont.)

On how many of the past 28 days ...	No days	1–5 days	6–12 days	13–15 days	16–22 days	23–27 days	Every day
9. Have you had a definite fear of losing control over eating?	0	1	2	3	4	5	6
10. Have you had a definite fear that you might gain weight?	0	1	2	3	4	5	6
11. Have you felt fat?	0	1	2	3	4	5	6
12. Have you had a strong desire to lose weight?	0	1	2	3	4	5	6

Questions 13–18: Please fill in the appropriate number in the boxes on the right. Remember that the questions only refer to the past 4 weeks (28 days).

Over the past 4 weeks (28 days) ...	
13. Over the past 28 days, how many *times* have you eaten what other people would regard as an *unusually large amount of food* (given the circumstances)?	_____
14. On how many of these days did you have a sense of having lost control over your eating (at the time that you were eating)?	_____
15. Over the past 28 days, on how many *days* have such episodes of overeating occurred (i.e., you have eaten an unusually large amount of food *and* have had a sense of loss of control at the time)?	_____
16. Over the past 28 days, how many *times* have you made yourself sick (vomit) as a means of controlling your shape or weight?	_____
17. Over the past 28 days, how many *times* have you taken laxatives as a means of controlling your shape or weight?	_____
18. Over the past 28 days, how many *times* have you exercised in a "driven" or "compulsive" way as a means of controlling your weight, shape or amount of fat, or to burn off calories?	_____

Questions 19–21: Please circle the appropriate number. *Please note that for these questions the term "binge eating" means* eating what others would regard as an unusually large amount of food for the circumstances, accompanied by a sense of having lost control over eating.

19. Over the past 28 days, on how many days have you eaten in secret (i.e., furtively)? ... Ignore episodes of binge eating	No days	1–5 days	6–12 days	13–15 days	16–22 days	23–27 days	Every day
	0	1	2	3	4	5	6

(cont.)

20. On what proportion of the times that you have eaten have you felt guilty (felt that you've done wrong) because of its effect on your shape or weight? ... Ignore episodes of binge eating	None of the time	A few of the times	Less than half	Half of the times	More than half	Most of the time	Every time
	0	1	2	3	4	5	6
21. Over the past 28 days, how concerned have you been about other people seeing you eat? ... Ignore episodes of binge eating	**Not at all**		**Slightly**		**Moderately**		**Markedly**
	0	1	2	3	4	5	6

Questions 22–28: Please circle the appropriate number on the right. Remember that the questions refer to the past 4 weeks (28 days) only.

On how many of the past 28 days ...	Not at all		Slightly		Moderately		Markedly
22. Has your *weight* influenced how you think about (judge) yourself as a person?	0	1	2	3	4	5	6
23. Has your *shape* influenced how you think about (judge) yourself as a person?	0	1	2	3	4	5	6
24. How much would it have upset you if you had been asked to weigh yourself once a week (no more, or less, often) for the next 4 weeks?	0	1	2	3	4	5	6
25. How dissatisfied have you been with your *weight*?	0	1	2	3	4	5	6
26. How dissatisfied have you been with your *shape*?	0	1	2	3	4	5	6
27. How uncomfortable have you felt seeing your body (for example, seeing your shape in the mirror, in a shop window reflection, while undressing or taking a bath or shower)?	0	1	2	3	4	5	6
28. How uncomfortable have you felt about *others* seeing your shape or figure (for example, in communal changing rooms, when swimming, or wearing tight clothes)?	0	1	2	3	4	5	6

What is your weight at present? (Please give your best estimate.) _____

What is your height? (Please give your best estimate.) _____

If female: Over the past 3–4 months have you missed any menstrual periods? _____

    If so, how many? _____

    Have you been taking the "pill"? _____

THANK YOU

APPENDIX B.3. CLINICAL IMPAIRMENT
ASSESSMENT QUESTIONNAIRE (CIA)

The Clinical Impairment Assessment Questionnaire (CIA) is a self-report instrument that was designed to be administered directly after the EDE-Q. The CIA provides information about the patient's impairment as a result of the eating disorder over the preceding 28 days. Impairment is assessed in the mood, cognitive, interpersonal, and work domains. Many clinicians find it useful to administer the EDE-Q and the CIA together at intake to aid clinical assessment and diagnosis. The EDE-Q and CIA also can be readministered mid-treatment or upon treatment completion to assess the patient's improvement over time.

Like the EDE-Q, the CIA is a self-report measure to be completed by the patient before treatment or between sessions. Instructions for the patient are provided on the CIA. Detailed scoring information and community norms are provided here with permission from its developers.

CIA SCORING INFORMATION

Introduction

The Clinical Impairment Assessment Questionnaire (CIA) is a 16-item self-report measure of the severity of psychosocial impairment resulting from eating disorder features (Bohn & Fairburn, 2008). It focuses on the past 28 days. The 16 items cover impairment in domains of life that are typically affected by eating disorder psychopathology: mood and self-perception, cognitive functioning, interpersonal functioning, and work performance. The purpose of the CIA is to provide a simple single index of the severity of psychosocial impairment secondary to eating disorder features.

The CIA is designed to be completed immediately after filling in the EDE-Q, which covers the same time frame. This ensures that patients have their eating disorder features "at the front of their mind" when filling in the CIA.

The CIA is intended to assist in the clinical assessment of the patient both before and after treatment.

Status

Tests of reliability, validity, sensitivity to change, and the instrument's ability to predict case status have been conducted, all of which support its use (Bohn et al., 2008).

Sources: Bohn, Doll, Cooper, O'Connor, Palmer, and Fairburn (2008) and Bohn and Fairburn (2008).

Scoring

Each item is rated on a Likert scale, with the response options being "Not at all," "A little," "Quite a bit," and "A lot." These responses are scored 0, 1, 2, and 3, respectively, with a higher rating indicating a higher level of impairment. Since it is the purpose of the CIA to measure the *overall severity* of secondary psychosocial impairment, a global CIA impairment score is calculated. To obtain the **global CIA impairment score,** the ratings on all items are added together with prorating of missing ratings, so long as at least 12 of the 16 items have been rated. The resulting score ranges from 0 to 48, with a higher score indicating a higher level of secondary psychosocial impairment. An ROC analysis showed that a global impairment score of 16 was the best cut-point for predicting eating disorder case status (Bohn et al., 2008).

FORM B.3. Clinical Impairment Assessment Questionnaire (CIA)

Copyright 2008 by Kristin Bohn and Christopher Fairburn

Instructions: Please place an "X" in the column which best describes how your eating habits, exercising, or feelings about your eating, shape or weight have affected your life over the past four weeks (28 days). Thank you.

	Over the past 28 days, to what extent have your ... eating habits ... exercising ... or feelings about your eating, shape or weight ...	Not at all	A little	Quite a bit	A lot
1	... made it difficult to concentrate?				
2	... made you feel critical of yourself?				
3	... stopped you going out with others?				
4	... affected your work performance (if applicable)?				
5	... made you forgetful?				
6	... affected your ability to make everyday decisions?				
7	... interfered with meals with family or friends?				
8	... made you upset?				
9	... made you feel ashamed of yourself?				
10	... made it difficult to eat out with others?				
11	... made you feel guilty?				
12	... interfered with you doing things you used to enjoy?				
13	... made you absent-minded?				
14	... made you feel like a failure?				
15	... interfered with your relationships with others?				
16	... made you worry?				

APPENDIX B.4. BODY IMAGE CHECKLIST

The Body Image Checklist is a self-report instrument used to ascertain the extent of body image disturbance. The Body Image Checklist queries the frequency of the patient's checking behaviors, avoidance strategies, and negative beliefs related to her appearance. The patient can complete this instrument at intake, just prior to starting body image interventions around session 14, or at both points. Scoring information and community norms are not available for the Body Image Checklist. However, the Body Image Checklist provides the therapist and patient with qualitative information about the presence and severity of the patient's body avoidance, checking, and dissatisfaction.

Responses on the Body Image Checklist are particularly useful for case conceptualization and during the third phase of treatment. The therapist should provide the patient with feedback about the extent of body checking and avoidance. Using the cognitive-behavioral model of eating disorders (see Figure 2.1), the therapist can remind the patient about how checking and avoidance behaviors negatively influence body image, cognitions, and eating disorder symptoms. During the third phase of treatment, the discontinuation of body checking will target those behaviors most endorsed by the patient on the Body Image Checklist. The patient's progress throughout treatment can also be tracked using this measure.

FORM B.4. Body Image Checklist

Instructions: Please answer these questions as they have applied to you over the PAST 4 WEEKS. Please place a check in the appropriate column.

Over the past 4 weeks ...	Not at all	Sometimes	Frequently	Not applicable
Questions about avoidance:				
Have you avoided seeing yourself in mirrors (or window reflections)?				
Have you avoided weighing yourself?				
Have you dressed in a way to disguise your appearance?				
Have you avoided your shape being seen by others (e.g., swimming pools, communal changing rooms)?				
Have you avoided taking part in physical activities because of your shape?				
Have you avoided shopping for clothes?				
Have you avoided being seen at home naked (e.g., when undressing or bathing)?				
Have you avoided wearing clothes that show the shape of your body?				
Have you avoided (or limited) close physical contact because of your dislike of your shape (e.g., shaking hands, sexual contact, hugging, kissing)?				
Have you avoided wearing clothes that show your skin (e.g., short-sleeve shirts, shorts)?				
Have you avoided social occasions because of your shape?				
Questions about checking:				
Have you studied your overall appearance in the mirror?				
Have you studied parts of your body in the mirror?				
Have you weighed yourself?				
Have you measured parts of your body?				
Have you assessed your size in other ways?				
Have you pinched yourself to see how much fat there is?				

(cont.)

Source: Cooper, Fairburn, and Hawker (2003).

From *Treatment Plans and Interventions for Bulimia and Binge-Eating Disorder* by Rene D. Zweig and Robert L. Leahy. Copyright 2012 by The Guilford Press. Permission to photocopy this form is granted to purchasers of this book for personal use only (see copyright page for details). This form may also be downloaded and printed from the book's page on The Guilford Press website.

Over the past 4 weeks ...	Not at all	Sometimes	Frequently	Not applicable
General questions:				
Have you felt unhappy about your shape?				
Have you worried about the size of particular parts of your body?				
Have you worried about your body wobbling?				
Have you felt ashamed or embarrassed about your body in public?				
Have you felt that other people were noticing your shape?				
Have you felt that your body was disgusting?				
Have you thought that other people were being critical of you because of your shape?				
Have you felt that you take up too much room (e.g., when sitting on sofa or bus seat)?				
Have you sought reassurance that your shape is not as bad as you think it is?				
Have people made critical comments about your shape or appearance?				

APPENDIX B.5. EATING DISORDER
BELIEF QUESTIONNAIRE (EDBQ)

The Eating Disorder Belief Questionnaire (EDBQ) is a self-report instrument that can be used to identify an adult or adolescent patient's thoughts, assumptions, and beliefs associated with weight, shape, and eating. The identification of these negative, recurring cognitions, which are common among patients with an eating disorder, will contribute to the case conceptualization and help guide the cognitive restructuring phase of treatment. The EDBQ demonstrates good reliability and validity. Thus, the therapist may use the EDBQ for research purposes and to evaluate cognitive change over the course of treatment. The therapist may choose to administer the EDBQ to the patient at treatment intake, prior to starting the second phase of treatment, and/or posttreatment.

The EDBQ is a self-report measure to be completed by the patient. Instructions for the patient are provided on the EDBQ. Scoring information is provided below to assist the therapist. After the patient completes the EDBQ, the therapist can calculate mean responses on each of the four factors by adding together the ratings for the relevant items and dividing the sum by the total number of items that contribute to that factor. The mean score for each factor can range from 0 to 100, with higher scores indicating the need for more cognitive restructuring in that area. Scores above 50, the mathematical median, on any particular factor indicate that a patient is particularly affected by and believes that category of beliefs. Community norms based on a large-scale sample are not available for the EDBQ. However, preliminary means were published for a small sample of adult females with BN and non-eating-disordered females (listed below). Patients with AN or BN exhibit stronger negative beliefs about shape and weight, eating, and the self than control females with no history of an eating disorder, and thus will have elevated scores on the EDBQ (Cooper & Hunt, 1998; Cooper & Turner, 2000).

Feedback about elevated scores can be given to the patient during orientation to treatment, and cognitive restructuring interventions should directly target the patient's most problematic beliefs. For example, a patient with a score of 72 on factor 4, control over eating, strongly believes that dietary restriction and compensatory mechanisms are necessary to control one's eating and weight. This belief should be included under Cognitive Factors on the patient's Case Conceptualization Worksheet. During treatment, cognitive restructuring and behavioral experiments should then target those cognitive beliefs most endorsed by the patient.

EDBQ SCORING INFORMATION

Items Loading on Each of the Four Factors

Factor 1: Negative self-beliefs
Negative core beliefs

Items: 1   3   4   5   11   13   17   22   27   29

Factor 2: Acceptance by others
Believes controlled weight and shape is necessary for acceptance by others

Items: 8   18   19   20   21   23   24   25   26   31

Factor 3: Self-acceptance
Believes controlled weight and shape is necessary for self-acceptance

Items: 2   7   9   12   30   32

Factor 4: Control over eating
Believes strict control over eating is necessary for self-control

Items: 6   10   14   15   16   28

Mean scores and standard deviations for females with BN (N = 12) and non-eating disordered controls (N = 18) (Cooper & Hunt, 1998):

	BN	Female controls
Factor 1:	67.3 (± 18.6)	12.7 (± 14.7)
Factor 2:	65.7 (± 21.5)	7.7 (± 9.4)
Factor 3:	92.7 (± 10.9)	43.3 (± 22.5)
Factor 4:	71.6 (± 19.8)	2.6 (± 4.3)

FORM B.5.   Eating Disorder Belief Questionnaire (EDBQ)

Instructions: Below are a series of items. Read each item carefully. Then choose a rating from the scale that best describes what you emotionally believe or feel, rather than what you rationally believe to be true. Choose the rating that best describes what you usually believe or what you believe most of the time. Write your rating in the space to the left of the item.

Rating Scale

0	10	20	30	40	50	60	70	80	90	100

I do not usually
believe this at all

I am usually completely
convinced that this is true

1. _____ I'm unlovable
2. _____ If my flesh is firm I'm more attractive
3. _____ I'm ugly
4. _____ I'm useless
5. _____ I'm a failure
6. _____ If I eat forbidden food I won't be able to stop
7. _____ If my stomach is flat I'll be more desirable
8. _____ If I lose weight I'll count more in the world
9. _____ If I eat desserts or puddings I'll get fat
10. _____ If I stay hungry I can guard against losing control and getting fat
11. _____ I'm all alone
12. _____ If I eat bad foods such as fats, sweets, bread and cereals they will turn into fat
13. _____ I'm no good
14. _____ If I eat normally I'll gain weight
15. _____ If I eat three meals a day like other people I'll gain weight
16. _____ If I've eaten something I have to get rid of it as soon as possible
17. _____ I'm not a likeable person
18. _____ If my hips are thin people will approve of me
19. _____ If I lose weight people will be friendly and want to get to know me
20. _____ If I gain weight it means I'm a bad person
21. _____ If my thighs are firm it means I'm a better person
22. _____ I don't like myself very much
23. _____ If I gain weight I'm nothing
24. _____ If my hips are narrow it means I'm successful
25. _____ If I lose weight people will care about me
26. _____ If my body shape is in proportion people will love me
27. _____ I'm dull
28. _____ If I binge and vomit I can stay in control
29. _____ I'm stupid
30. _____ If my body is lean I can feel good about myself
31. _____ If my bottom is small people will take me seriously
32. _____ Body fat/flabbiness is disgusting

Source: Cooper, Cohen-Tovée, Todd, Wells, and Tovée (1997).

From *Treatment Plans and Interventions for Bulimia and Binge-Eating Disorder* by Rene D. Zweig and Robert L. Leahy. Copyright 2012 by The Guilford Press. Permission to photocopy this form is granted to purchasers of this book for personal use only (see copyright page for details). This form may also be downloaded and printed from the book's page on The Guilford Press website.

APPENDIX B.6. BODY MASS INDEX (BMI)

Body mass index (BMI) is a simple calculation often used to classify body weight. By taking an individual's height into account [BMI = weight (in kg)/height^2 (in m^2)], BMI provides a single number that can be compared across individuals and genders and over time. Although not a perfect tool, BMI is valuable for defining healthy weights (BMI of 19–24), underweight (BMI $\leq$ 18), overweight (BMI $\geq$ 25), obesity (BMI $\geq$ 30), and morbid obesity (BMI $\geq$ 40). Body weight and BMI are typically evaluated upon intake and throughout the course of treatment. These charts are also useful for discussing normal weight ranges with patients and their families. Separate charts are provided for adults and adolescents.

FORM B.6. Body Mass Index (BMI) Table for Adult Men and Women

| | Underweight | | | | Normal | | | | | Overweight | | | | | Obese | | | | | |
BMI	16	17	18	19	20	21	22	23	24	25	26	27	28	29	30	31	32	33	34	35
Height										*Body weight (pounds)*										
4'10"	77	82	86	91	96	100	105	110	115	119	124	129	134	138	143	148	153	158	162	167
4'11"	79	84	89	94	99	104	109	114	119	124	128	133	138	143	148	153	158	163	168	173
5'	82	87	92	97	102	107	112	118	123	128	133	138	143	148	153	158	163	168	174	179
5'1"	85	90	96	100	106	111	116	122	127	132	137	143	148	153	158	164	169	174	180	185
5'2"	88	93	99	104	109	115	120	126	131	136	142	147	153	158	164	169	175	180	186	191
5'3"	91	96	102	107	113	118	124	130	135	141	146	152	158	163	169	175	180	186	191	197
5'4"	93	99	105	110	116	122	128	134	140	145	151	157	163	169	174	180	186	192	197	204
5'5"	96	102	108	114	120	126	132	138	144	150	156	162	168	174	180	186	192	198	204	210
5'6"	99	106	112	118	124	130	136	142	148	155	161	167	173	179	186	192	198	204	210	216
5'7"	102	109	115	121	127	134	140	146	153	159	166	172	178	185	191	198	204	211	217	223
5'8"	105	112	119	125	131	138	144	151	158	164	171	177	184	190	197	203	210	216	223	230
5'9"	109	115	122	128	135	142	149	155	162	169	176	182	189	196	203	209	216	223	230	236
5'10"	112	119	126	132	139	146	153	160	167	174	181	188	195	202	209	216	222	229	236	243
5'11"	115	122	129	136	143	150	157	165	172	179	186	193	200	208	215	222	229	236	243	250
6'	118	125	133	140	147	154	162	169	177	184	191	199	206	213	221	228	235	242	250	258
6'1"	121	129	137	144	151	159	166	174	182	189	197	204	212	219	227	235	242	250	257	265
6'2"	125	133	140	148	155	163	171	179	186	194	202	210	218	225	233	241	249	257	264	272
6'3"	128	136	144	152	160	168	176	184	192	200	208	216	224	232	240	248	256	264	272	279

Source: National Heart, Lung, and Blood Institute, a part of the National Institutes of Health and the U.S. Department of Health and Human Services.

From *Treatment Plans and Interventions for Bulimia and Binge-Eating Disorder* by Rene D. Zweig and Robert L. Leahy. Copyright 2012 by The Guilford Press. Permission to photocopy this form is granted to purchasers of this book for personal use only (see copyright page for details). This form may also be downloaded and printed from the book's page on The Guilford Press website.

BMI is age- and sex-specific for children and teens. To determine whether a child or teen is at a healthy weight:

1. Obtain an accurate height and weight measurement.
2. Calculate the child's BMI using the online calculator at *apps.nccd.cdc.gov/dnpabmi.*
3. Determine the BMI-for-age percentile using Forms B.7a and B.7b.
4. Evaluate whether the child's/teen's BMI-for-age percentile falls within the healthy range.

Underweight:	< 5th percentile
Normal weight:	5th–85th percentile
Overweight:	85th–95th percentile
Obese:	≥ 95th percentile

Source: Centers for Disease Control and Prevention.

FORM B.7A. Body Weight for Adolescent Boys

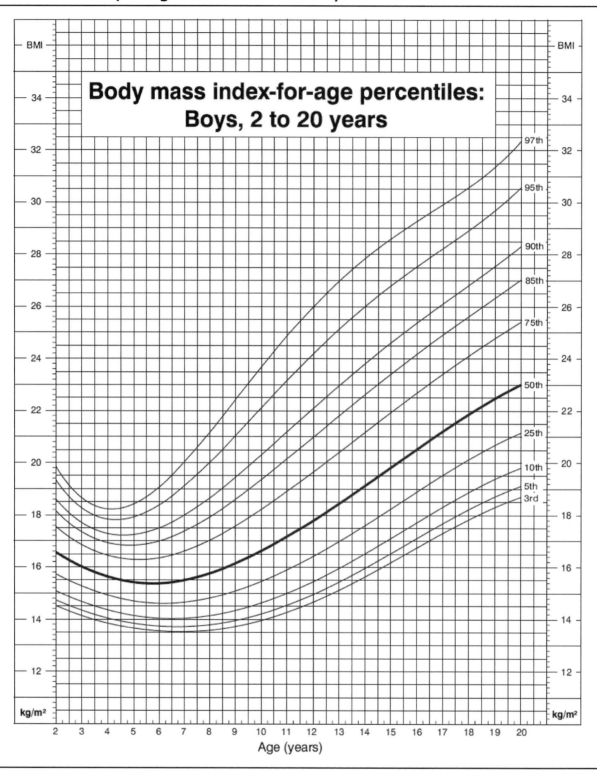

Body mass index-for-age percentiles: Boys, 2 to 20 years

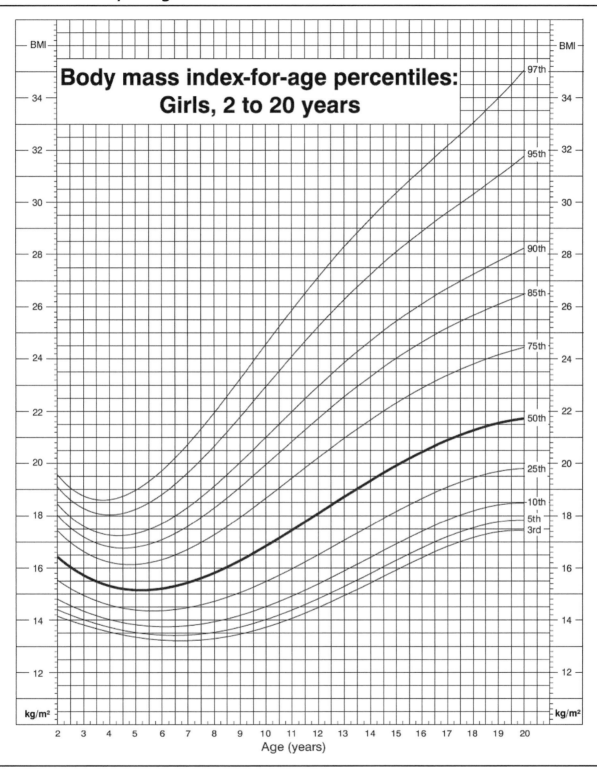

APPENDIX B.8. EVALUATION OF SUICIDE RISK

The final included assessment measure assists therapists in evaluating the degree of suicidality and the presence of suicide risk factors. The Evaluation of Suicide Risk is included because depression and suicidality commonly co-occur with eating disorders. Whenever a patient reports significant clinical depression, hopelessness, or suicidal ideation, the therapist can use the Evaluation of Suicide Risk to query about risk factors and, when present, to develop a safety plan collaboratively with the patient.

The Evaluation of Suicide Risk assesses a variety thoughts, behaviors, and past actions that put an individual at increased risk for self-harm. A greater number of positive responses on the Evaluation of Suicide Risk, especially if the thoughts or intent are current, indicates a greater risk of self-harm. In particular, hopelessness, at least one prior suicide attempt, alcoholism or substance abuse, a friend or family member's past attempted or completed suicide, and male gender are associated with an elevated risk of suicide (Beck, Brown, Berchick, Stewart, & Steer, 1990; Thompson & Light, 2011). If a patient reports any current intent for suicide, a current plan for self-harm, few reasons for living, and/or access to a weapon or other means of suicidal injury, the therapist should consider immediate hospitalization to ensure the patient's safety. It is best if hospitalization is agreed upon by both patient and therapist. However, hospitalization without the patient's consent is possible and advisable when there is any imminent intent of self-harm. If the therapist is sufficiently concerned about the risk for suicide (e.g., few reasons for living, a history of suicide attempts, and hopelessness), but in the absence of a current plan or other indication of immediate intent requiring hospitalization, the therapist should develop a written safety contract with the patient. A sample safety contract is provided at the end of the Evaluation of Suicide Risk. The safety contract should be accompanied by an increase in the frequency of outpatient psychotherapy sessions and/or a referral to a psychopharmacologist for antidepressant medication.

FORM B.8. Evaluation of Suicide Risk

Patient's name: _____   Date: _____

Therapist's name: _____

Evaluate for current suicidal ideation and behavior and for past incidence of suicidal plans, intentions, or behavior.

Questions	Current	Past
Do you have thoughts of harming yourself? [If yes:] Describe.		
Have you ever felt indifferent about whether something dangerous would happen to you and you took a lot of risk—like you really didn't care if you died or hurt yourself? [If yes:] Describe.		
Have you ever threatened that you would hurt yourself? [If yes:] Whom did you say this to? Why?		
Have you ever tried to hurt yourself on purpose? [If no, go on to p. 3 of form]		
Exactly what did you do to try to hurt yourself?		
How many times have you tried this? When? Describe.		

(cont.)

Questions	Current	Past
Had you planned to hurt yourself, or was it spontaneous?		
What was your state of mind when you attempted to hurt yourself? Were you depressed, spaced out, anxious, relieved, angry, excited? Were you using alcohol, medication, other drugs?		
Did you call someone at that time, or were you discovered by someone? What happened?		
Did you go to a doctor or to the hospital? [Obtain release of information.]		
Did you feel glad that you were alive? Embarrassed? Guilty? Sorry you didn't kill yourself?		
Did you want to hurt yourself soon after your attempt?		
Was there any event that triggered your attempt? [If no, go to next page of form]		
What were you thinking after this event that made you want to hurt yourself?		

(cont.)

Questions	Current	Past
If something like that happened again, how would you handle it?		
Has any family member or close friend ever hurt him- or herself?		
How would you describe your current [past] desire to live? None, weak, moderate, or strong?		
How would you describe your current [past] desire to die? None, weak, moderate, or strong?		
[If current or past desire to die:] What would be the reason for wanting to die or harm yourself? Hopelessness, depression, revenge, getting rid of anxiety, being with a lost loved one again, other reasons?		
[If current or past desire to die:] Have you ever planned to hurt yourself? What was the plan? Why did you [did you not] carry it out?		
Are there any reasons why you would *not* harm yourself? Explain.		
Do you have more reasons to live than to die?		

(cont.)

Questions	Current	Past
[If not:] What would have to change so that you would want to live more?		
Do you own a weapon?		
Do you live on a high floor or near a high bridge?		
Are you saving medications for a future attempt to hurt yourself?		
Do you drive excessively fast?		
Do you drink more than three glasses of liquor or beer a day? Do you use any medications? Other drugs? Do these substances affect your mood? [If yes:] How?		
Have you written a suicide note? Have you recently written out a will?		
Do you feel there is any hope that things can get better?		
What are the reasons why things could be hopeful?		

(cont.)

Questions	Current	Past
Why would things seem hopeless?		
Would you be willing to promise me that you would not do anything to harm yourself until you have called me and spoken with me?		
Is your promise a solemn promise that I can rely on, or do you have doubts about whether you can keep this promise? [If doubts:] What are these doubts?		
Can I speak with [loved ones or close friend] to be sure that we have all the support that we need?		
[Does this patient need to be hospitalized? Increase frequency of treatment contact and level or type of medication? ECT?]		

Therapist: Summarize dates, precipitating factors, and nature of the patient's previous suicide attempts, if any:

_____

_____

_____

_____

_____

If the patient is willing to promise that she/he will contact and speak with the therapist before engaging in any self-harmful action, have her/him sign this statement:

I, _____, promise that I will not do anything to harm myself until I have called and spoken to you, my therapist. In the event that I cannot reach my therapist, I agree to call 9-1-1 or go to my nearest emergency room immediately. I also agree that you may speak with a loved one or close friend of mine to be sure that you and I have all the support we need.

_____   _____
Patient's signature   Therapist's signature

_____
Date

Recommended Additional Reading

PSYCHOEDUCATION FOR PATIENTS AND THEIR FAMILIES

The Body Image Workbook: An Eight-Step Program for Learning to Like Your Looks (2nd ed.) by Thomas F. Cash. Oakland, CA: New Harbinger, 2008.

Eating Disorders by National Institute of Mental Health. *www.nimh.nih.gov/health/publications/eating-disorders/nimheatingdisorders.pdf.*

Feeling Good about the Way You Look: A Program for Overcoming Body Image Problems by Sabine Wilhelm. New York: Guilford Press, 2006.

Help Your Teenager Beat an Eating Disorder by James Lock and Daniel le Grange. New York: Guilford Press, 2005.

Never Good Enough: Freeing Yourself from the Chains of Perfectionism by Monica Ramirez Basco. New York: Free Press, 1999.

Overcoming Binge Eating by Christopher G. Fairburn. New York: Guilford Press, 1995.

RESOURCES FOR THERAPISTS

Assessment of Eating Disorders edited by James E. Mitchell and Carol B. Peterson. New York: Guilford Press, 2005.

Body Image: A Handbook of Science, Practice, and Prevention (2nd ed.) edited by Thomas F. Cash and Linda Smolak. New York: Guilford Press, 2011.

Eating Disorders: A Guide to Medical Care and Complications (2nd ed.) by Philip S. Mehler and Arnold E. Anderson. Baltimore: Johns Hopkins University Press, 2010.

Eating Disorders and Obesity: A Comprehensive Handbook (2nd ed.) edited by Christopher G. Fairburn and Kelly D. Brownell. New York: Guilford Press, 2005.

Handbook of Treatment for Eating Disorders (2nd ed.) edited by David M. Garner and Paul E. Garfinkel. New York: Guilford Press, 1997.

The Treatment of Eating Disorders: A Clinical Handbook edited by Carlos M. Grilo and James E. Mitchell. New York: Guilford Press, 2010.

PROFESSIONAL ORGANIZATIONS AND USEFUL WEBSITES

Academy for Eating Disorders (AED)
www.aedweb.org

Academy of Cognitive Therapy (ACT)
www.academyofct.org

Association for Behavioral and Cognitive Therapies (ABCT)
www.abct.org

Body Mass Index Calculator
www.nhlbisupport.com/bmi

British Association for Behavioural and Cognitive Psychotherapies (BABCP)
www.babcp.com

Centers for Disease Control and Prevention
www.cdc.gov/healthyweight

International Association of Eating Disorders Professionals (IAEDP)
www.iaedp.com

MyPlate
www.choosemyplate.gov

National Eating Disorders Association (NEDA)
www.nationaleatingdisorders.org

Something Fishy
www.something-fishy.org

BACKGROUND BOOKS IN COGNITIVE–BEHAVIORAL THERAPY

Anxiety Free: Unravel Your Fears before They Unravel You by Robert L. Leahy. New York: Hay House, 2009.
Beat the Blues Before They Beat You: How to Overcome Your Depression by Robert L. Leahy. New York: Hay House, 2010.
Clinician's Guide to Mind Over Mood by Christine A. Padesky and Dennis Greenberger. New York: Guilford Press, 1995.
Cognitive Behavior Therapy: Basics and Beyond (2nd ed.) by Judith S. Beck. New York: Guilford Press, 2011.
Cognitive Therapy of Depression by Aaron T. Beck, A. John Rush, Brian F. Shaw, and Gary Emery. New York: Guilford Press, 1979.
Cognitive Therapy Techniques: A Practitioner's Guide by Robert L. Leahy. New York: Guilford Press, 2003.
The Feeling Good Handbook by David D. Burns. New York: Penguin, 1999.
Mind Over Mood: Change How You Feel by Changing the Way You Think by Dennis Greenberger and Christine A. Padesky. New York: Guilford Press, 1995.
Treatment Plans and Interventions for Depression and Anxiety Disorders (2nd ed.) by Robert L. Leahy, Stephen J. F. Holland, and Lata K. McGinn. New York: Guilford Press, 2012.

References

Agras, W. S. (1997). Pharmacotherapy of bulimia nervosa and binge eating disorder: Longer-term outcomes. *Psychopharmacological Bulletin, 33,* 433–436.

Agras, W. S. (2001). The consequences and costs of the eating disorders. *Psychiatric Clinics of North America, 24,* 371–379.

Agras, W. S., Crow, S. J., Halmi, K. A., Mitchell, J. E., Wilson, G. T., & Kraemer, H. C. (2000). Outcome predictors for the cognitive behavior treatment of bulimia nervosa: Data from a multisite study. *American Journal of Psychiatry, 157,* 1302–1308.

Agras, W. S., Rossiter, E. M., Arnow, B., Schneider, J. A., Telch, C. F., Raeburn, S. D., et al. (1992). Pharmacologic and cognitive-behavioral treatment for bulimia nervosa. *American Journal of Psychiatry, 149,* 82–87.

Agras, W. S., Walsh, B. T., Fairburn, C. G., Wilson, G. T., & Kraemer, H. C. (2000). A multicenter comparison of cognitive-behavioral therapy and interpersonal psychotherapy for bulimia nervosa. *Archives of General Psychiatry, 57,* 459–466.

Alvarenga, M. S., Scagliusi, F. B., & Philippi, S. T. (2008). Changing attitudes, beliefs and feelings towards food in bulimic patients. *Archivos Latinoamericanos de Nutricion, 58,* 274–279.

American Psychiatric Association. (2000). *Diagnostic and statistical manual of mental disorders* (4th ed., text rev.). Washington, DC: Author.

American Psychiatric Association. (2006). *Practice guideline for the treatment of patients with eating disorders* (3rd ed.). Washington, DC: Author.

Anderson, A. E. (1992). Medical complications of eating disorders. In J. Yager, H. E. Gwirtsman, & C. K. Edelstein (Eds.), *Special problems in managing eating disorders* (pp. 119–144). Washington, DC: American Psychiatric Press.

Arcelus, J., Whight, D., Langham, C., Baggott, J., McGrain, L., Meadows, L., et al. (2009). A case series evaluation of a modified version of interpersonal psychotherapy (IPT) for the treatment of bulimic eating disorders: A pilot study. *European Eating Disorders Review, 17,* 260–268.

Beck, A. T., Brown, G., Berchick, R. J., Stewart, B. L., & Steer, R. A. (1990). Relationship between hopelessness and ultimate suicide: A replication with psychiatric outpatients. *American Journal of Psychiatry, 147,* 190–195.

Beck, A. T., Rush, A. J., Shaw, B. F., & Emery, G. (1979). *Cognitive therapy of depression.* New York: Guilford Press.

Beck, A. T., & Steer, R. A. (1993). *Beck Anxiety Inventory manual.* San Antonio, TX: Psychological Corporation.

Beck, A. T., Steer, R. A., & Brown, G. K. (1996). *Manual for Beck Depression Inventory II.* San Antonio, TX: Psychological Corporation.

Beck, J. S. (2011). *Cognitive behavior therapy: Basics and beyond* (2nd ed.). New York: Guilford Press.

Becker, A. E., Grinspoon, S. K., Klibanski, A., & Herzog, D. B. (1999). Eating disorders. *New England Journal of Medicine, 340,* 1092–1098.

Bohn, K., Doll, D. A., Cooper, Z., O'Connor, M. E., Palmer, R. L., & Fairburn, C. G. (2008). The measurement of impairment due to eating disorder psychopathology. *Behaviour Research and Therapy, 46,* 1105–1110.

Bohn, K., & Fairburn, C. G. (2008). Clinical Impairment Assessment Questionnaire (CIA 3.0). In C. G. Fairburn, *Cognitive behavior therapy and eating disorders* (pp. 315–317). New York: Guilford Press.

Braun, D. L., Sunday, S. R., & Halmi, K. A. (1994). Psychiatric comorbidity in patients with eating disorders. *Psychological Medicine, 24,* 859–867.

Brewerton, T. D., Lydiard, R. B., Herzog, D. B., Brotman, A. W., O'Neil, P. M., & Ballenger, J. C. (1995). Comorbidity of Axis I psychiatric disorders in bulimia nervosa. *Journal of Clinical Psychiatry, 56,* 77–80.

Bulik, C. M., Sullivan, P. F., Carter, F. A., & Joyce, R. R. (1997). Lifetime comorbidity of alcohol dependence in women with bulimia nervosa. *Addictive Behaviors, 22,* 437–446.

Bulik, C. M., Tozzi, F., Anderson, C., Mazzeo, S. E., Aggen, S., & Sullivan, P. F. (2003). The relationship between eating disorders and components of perfectionism. *American Journal of Psychiatry, 160,* 366–368.

Button, E. J., Benson, E., Nollett, C., & Palmer, R. L. (2005). Don't forget EDNOS (eating disorder not otherwise specified): Patterns of service use in an eating disorders service. *Psychiatric Bulletin, 29,* 134–136.

Byrne, S. M., & McLean, N. J. (2002). The cognitive-behavioral model of bulimia nervosa: A direct evaluation. *International Journal of Eating Disorders, 31,* 17–31.

Carter, J. C., Olmsted, M. P., Kaplan, A. S., McCabe, R. E., Mills, J. S., & Aimé, A. (2003). Self-help for bulimia nervosa: A randomized controlled trial. *American Journal of Psychiatry, 160,* 973–978.

Cash, T. F., & Deagle, E. A. (1997). The nature and extent of body-image disturbances in anorexia nervosa and bulimia nervosa: A meta-analysis. *International Journal of Eating Disorders, 22,* 107–125.

Cash, T. F., & Henry, P. E. (1995). Women's body images: The results of a national survey in the U.S.A. *Sex Roles, 33,* 19–28.

Cooper, M., Cohen-Tovée, E., Todd, G., Wells, A., & Tovée, M. (1997). The Eating Disorder Belief Questionnaire: Preliminary development. *Behaviour Research and Therapy, 35,* 381–388.

Cooper, M., & Hunt, J. (1998). Core beliefs and underlying assumptions in bulimia nervosa and depression. *Behaviour Research and Therapy, 36,* 895–898.

Cooper, M., & Turner, H. (2000). Underlying assumptions and core beliefs in anorexia nervosa and dieting. *British Journal of Clinical Psychology, 39,* 215–218.

Cooper, M. J., Fairburn, C. G., & Hawker, D. M. (2003). *Cognitive-behavioral treatment of obesity.* New York: Guilford Press.

Cooper, M. J., Todd, G., & Wells, A. (2000). *Bulimia nervosa: A cognitive therapy programme for clients.* London: Jessica Kingsley.

Cooper, M. J., Wells, A., & Todd, G. (2004). A cognitive model of bulimia nervosa. *British Journal of Clinical Psychology, 43,* 1–16.

Corcos, M., Taïeb, O., Benoit-Lamy, S., Paterniti, S., Jeammet, P., & Flament, M. F. (2002). Suicide attempts in women with bulimia nervosa: Frequency and characteristics. *Acta Psychiatrica Scandinavica, 106,* 381–386.

Deaver, C. M., Miltenberger, R. G., Smyth, J., Meidinger, A., & Crosby, R. (2003). An evaluation of affect and binge eating. *Behavior Modification, 27,* 578–599.

Eating Disorders Work Group, American Psychiatric Association. (2010, October 6). *Eating Disorders.* Retrieved from *www.dsm5.org/ProposedRevisions/Pages/Default.aspx.*

Eisler, I., Dare, C., Russell, G. F., Szmukler, G., le Grange, D., & Dodge, E. (1997). Family and individual therapy for anorexia nervosa: A 5-year follow-up. *Archives of General Psychiatry, 54,* 1025–1030.

Esplen, M. J., Garfinkel, P. E., Olmsted, M., Gallop, R. M., & Kennedy, S. (1998). A randomized controlled trial of guided imagery in bulimia nervosa. *Psychological Medicine, 28,* 1347–1357.

Fairburn, C. G. (1997). Interpersonal psychotherapy for bulimia nervosa. In D. M. Garner & P. E. Garfinkel (Eds.), *Handbook of treatment for eating disorders* (2nd ed.), (pp. 278–294). New York: Guilford Press.

Fairburn, C. G., Agras, W. S., Walsh, B. T., Wilson, G. T., & Stice, E. (2004). Prediction of outcome in bulimia nervosa by early change in treatment. *American Journal of Psychiatry, 161,* 2322–2324.

Fairburn, C. G., & Beglin, S. J. (2008). Eating Disorder Examination Questionnaire (EDE-Q 6.0). In C. G. Fairburn, *Cognitive behavior therapy and eating disorders* (pp. 309–313). New York: Guilford Press.

Fairburn, C. G., & Cooper, Z. (1993). The Eating Disorder Examination (12th edition). In C. G. Fairburn & G. T. Wilson (Eds.), *Binge eating: Nature, assessment, and treatment* (pp. 317–360). New York: Guilford Press.

Fairburn, C. G., Cooper, Z., Bohn, K., O'Connor, M. E., Doll, H. A., & Palmer, R. L. (2007). The severity and status of eating disorder NOS: Implications for DSM-V. *Behaviour Research and Therapy, 45,* 1705–1715.

Fairburn, C. G., Cooper, Z., & Cooper, P. J. (1986). The clinical features and maintenance of bulimia nervosa. In K. D. Brownell & J. P. Foreyt (Eds.), *Handbook of eating disorders: Physiology, psychology, and treatment of obesity, anorexia, and bulimia* (pp. 389–404). New York: Basic Books.

Fairburn, C. G., Cooper, Z., Doll, H. A., Norman, P., & O'Connor, M. (2000). The natural course of bulimia nervosa and binge eating disorder in young women. *Archives of General Psychiatry, 57,* 659–665.

Fairburn, C. G., Cooper, Z., Doll, H. A., O'Connor, M. E., Bohn, K., Hawker, D. M., et al. (2009). Transdiagnostic cognitive-behavioral therapy for patients with eating disorders: A two-site trial with 60-week follow-up. *American Journal of Psychiatry, 166,* 311–319.

Fairburn, C. G., Cooper, Z., & Shafran, R. (2003). Cognitive behaviour therapy for eating disorders: A "transdiagnostic" theory and treatment. *Behaviour Research and Therapy, 41,* 509–528.

Fairburn, C. G., & Harrison, P. J. (2003). Eating disorders. *Lancet, 361,* 407–416.

Fairburn, C. G., Jones, R., Peveler, R. C., Carr, S. J., Solomon, R. A., O'Connor, et al. (1991). Three psychological treatments for bulimia nervosa: A comparative trial. *Archives of General Psychiatry, 48,* 463–469.

Fairburn, C. G., Marcus, M. D., & Wilson, G. T. (1993). Cognitive-behavioral therapy for binge eating and bulimia nervosa: A comprehensive treatment manual. In C. G. Fairburn & G. T. Wilson (Eds.), *Binge eating: Nature, assessment, and treatment* (pp. 361–404). New York: Guilford Press.

Fairburn, C. G., Norman, P. A., Welch, S. L., O'Connor, M. E., Doll, H. A., & Peveler, R. C. (1995). A prospective study of outcome in bulimia nervosa and the long-term effects of three psychological treatments. *Archives of General Psychiatry, 52,* 304–312.

Fairburn, C. G., Welch, S. L., Doll, H. A., Davies, B. A., & O'Connor, M. E. (1997). Risk factors for bulimia nervosa: A community-based case-control study. *Archives of General Psychiatry, 54,* 509–517.

Favaro, A., & Santonastaso, P. (1999). Different types of self-injurious behavior in bulimia nervosa. *Comprehensive Psychiatry, 40,* 57–60.

Fichter, M. M., Quadflieg, N., & Hedlund, S. (2008). Long-term course of binge eating disorder and bulimia nervosa: Relevance for nosology and diagnostic criteria. *International Journal of Eating Disorders, 41,* 577–586.

Fink, E. L., Smith, A. R., Gordon, K. H., Holm-Denoma, J. M., & Joiner, T. E., Jr. (2009). Psychological correlates of purging disorder as compared with other eating disorders: An exploratory investigation. *International Journal of Eating Disorders, 42,* 31–39.

Franko, D. L., Keel, P. K., Dorer, D. J., Blais, M. A., Delinsky, S. S., Eddy, K. T., et al. (2004). What predicts suicide attempts in women with eating disorders? *Psychological Medicine, 34,* 843–853.

Frederick, D. A., Peplau, L. A., & Lever, J. (2006). The swimsuit issue: Correlates of body image in a sample of 52,677 heterosexual adults. *Body Image, 3,* 413–419.

Helverskov, J. L., Clausen, L., Mors, O., Frydenberg, M., Thomsen, P. H., & Rokkedal, K. (2010). Transdiagnostic outcome of eating disorders: A 30-month follow-up study of 629 patients. *European Eating Disorders Review, 18,* 453–463.

Hendricks, P. S., & Thompson, K. (2005). An integration of cognitive-behavioral therapy and interpersonal psychotherapy for bulimia nervosa: A case study using the case formulation method. *International Journal of Eating Disorders, 37,* 171–174.

Holderness, C. C., Brooks-Gunn, J., & Warren, M. P. (1994). Co-morbidity of eating disorders and substance abuse: Review of the literature. *International Journal of Eating Disorders, 16,* 1–34.

Hudson, J. I., Hiripi, E., Pope, H. G., Jr., & Kessler, R. C. (2007). The prevalence and correlates of eating disorders in the National Comorbidity Survey Replication. *Biological Psychiatry, 61,* 348–358.

Kabat-Zinn, J. (1990). *Full catastrophe living: Using the wisdom of your body and mind to face stress, pain, and illness* (pp. 53–58). New York: Dell.

Kassett, J. A., Gershon, E. S., Maxwell, M. E., Guroff, J. J., Kazuba, D. M., Smith, A. L., et al. (1989). Psychiatric disorders in the first-degree relatives of probands with bulimia nervosa. *American Journal of Psychiatry, 146,* 1468–1471.

Kaye, W. H., Bulik, C. M., Thornton, R., Barbarich, N., Masters, K., & Price Foundation Collaborative Group. (2004). Comorbidity of anxiety disorders with anorexia and bulimia nervosa. *American Journal of Psychiatry, 161,* 2215–2221.

Kaye, W. H., Devlin, B., Barbarich, N., Bulik, C. M., Thornton, L., Bacanu, S. A., et al. (2004). Genetic analysis of bulimia nervosa: Methods and sample description. *International Journal of Eating Disorders, 35,* 556–570.

Kaye, W. H., Weltzin, T. E., Hsu, L. K., McConaha, C. W., & Bolton, B. (1993). Amount of calories retained after binge eating and vomiting. *American Journal of Psychiatry, 150,* 969–971.

Keel, P. K. (2007). Purging disorder: Subthreshold variant or full-threshold eating disorder? *International Journal of Eating Disorders, 40,* S89–S94.

Keel, P. K., & Mitchell, J. E. (1997). Outcome in bulimia nervosa. *American Journal of Psychiatry, 154,* 313–321.

Keel, P. K., Mitchell, J. E., Miller, K. B., Davis, R. L., & Crow, S. J. (1999). Long-term outcome of bulimia nervosa. *Archives of General Psychiatry, 56,* 63–69.

Kendler, K. S., MacLean, C., Neale, M., Kessler, R., Heath, A., & Eaves, L. (1991). The genetic epidemiology of bulimia nervosa. *American Journal of Psychiatry, 148,* 1627–1637.

Latner, J. D., & Clyne, C. (2008). The diagnostic validity of the criteria for binge eating disorder. *International Journal of Eating Disorders, 41,* 1–14.

le Grange, D., Crosby, R. D., Rathouz, P. J., & Leventhal, B. L. (2007). A randomized controlled comparison of family-based treatment and supportive psychotherapy for adolescent bulimia nervosa. *Archives of General Psychiatry, 64,* 1049–1056.

le Grange, D., & Lock, J. (2009). *Treating bulimia in adolescents: A family-based approach.* New York: Guilford Press.

Leahy, R. L. (2003). *Cognitive therapy techniques: A practitioner's guide.* New York: Guilford Press.

Leahy, R. L. (2005). *The worry cure: Seven steps to stop worry from stopping you.* New York: Guilford Press.

Leahy, R. L. (2002). A model of emotional schemas. *Cognitive and Behavioral Practice, 9,* 177–190.

Leahy, R. L., & Holland, S. J. (2000). *Treatment plans and interventions for depression and anxiety disorders* (pp. 260–264). New York: Guilford Press.

Leahy, R. L., Holland, S. J. F., & McGinn, L. K. (2012). *Treatment plans and interventions for depression and anxiety disorders* (2nd ed.). New York: Guilford Press.

Leahy, R. L., Tirch, D., & Napolitano, L. (2012). *Emotion regulation in psychotherapy: A practitioner's guide.* New York: Guilford Press.

Lewandowski, L. M., Gebing, T. A., Anthony, T. L., & O'Brien, W. H. (1997). Meta-analysis of cognitive-behavioral treatment studies for bulimia. *Clinical Psychology Review, 17,* 703–718.

Machado, P. P., Machado, B. C., Gonçalves, S., & Hoek, H. W. (2007). The prevalence of eating disorders not otherwise specified. *International Journal of Eating Disorders, 40,* 212–217.

Marlatt, G. A., & Witkiewitz, K. (2005). Relapse prevention for alcohol and drug problems. In G. A. Marlatt & D. M. Donovan (Eds.), *Relapse prevention: Maintenance strategies in the treatment of addictive disorders* (pp. 1–44). New York: Guilford Press.

McElroy, S. L., Arnold, L. M., Shapira, N. A., Keck, P. E., Jr., Rosenthal, N. R., Karim, M. R., et al. (2003). Topiramate in the treatment of binge eating disorder associated with obesity: A randomized, placebo-controlled trial. *American Journal of Psychiatry, 160,* 255–261.

Meads, C., Gold, L., & Burls, A. (2001). How effective is outpatient care compared to inpatient care for the treatment of anorexia nervosa? A systematic review. *European Eating Disorders Review, 9,* 229–241.

Mehler, P. S., & Anderson, A. E. (2000). *Eating disorders: A guide to medical care and complications.* Baltimore, MD: Johns Hopkins University Press.

Mehler, P. S., Birmingham, L. C., Crow, S. J., & Jahraus, J. P. (2010). Medical complications of eating disorders. In C. M. Grilo & J. E. Mitchell (Eds.), *The treatment of eating disorders: A clinical handbook* (pp. 66–80). New York: Guilford Press.

Mitchell, J. E., Agras, S., & Wonderlich, S. (2007). Treatment of bulimia nervosa: Where are we and where are we going? *International Journal of Eating Disorders, 40,* 95–101.

Mitchell, J. E., Pyle, R. L., Eckert, E. D., Hatsukami, D., Pomeroy, C., & Zimmerman, R. (1990). A comparison study of antidepressents and structured intensive group psychotherapy in the treatment of bulimia nervosa. *Archives of General Psychiatry, 47,* 149–157.

National Institute for Clinical Excellence. (2004). *Eating disorders: Core interventions in the treatment and management of anorexia nervosa, bulimia nervosa and related eating disorders* (National Clinical Practice Guideline Number 9). London: British Psychological Society and Gaskell.

New Avenues. (2009). *Guidelines to use of Axis V: Global Assessment Functioning scale.* Retrieved July 21, 2011, from *www.newavenuesonline.com/provider/forms/getpdf.aspx?id=45.*

Patton, G. C., Selzer, R., Coffrey, C., Carlin, J. B., & Wolfe, R. (1999). Onset of adolescent eating disorders: Population based cohort study over 3 years. *British Medical Journal, 318,* 765–768.

Pompili, M., Girardi, P., Tatarelli, G., Ruberto, A., & Tatarelli, R. (2006). Suicide and attempted suicide in eating disorders, obesity and weight-image concern. *Eating Behaviors, 7,* 384–394.

Reas, D. L., & Grilo, C. M. (2008). Review and meta-analysis of pharmacotherapy for binge-eating disorder. *Obesity, 16,* 2024–2038.

Reas, D. L., Williamson, D. A., Martin, C. K., & Zucker, N. L. (2000). Duration of illness predicts outcome for bulimia nervosa: A long-term follow-up study. *International Journal of Eating Disorders, 27,* 428–434.

Ricca, V., Mannucci, E., Mezzani, B., Di Bernardo, M., Zucchi, T., Paionni, A., et al. (2001). Psychopathological and clinical features of outpatients with an eating disorder not otherwise specified. *Eating and Weight Disorders, 6,* 157–165.

Roberto, C. A., Steinglass, J., Mayer, L. E. S., Attia, E., & Walsh, B. T. (2008). The clinical significance of amenorrhea as a diagnostic criterion for anorexia nervosa. *International Journal of Eating Disorders, 41,* 559–563.

Rodin, J., Silberstein, L. R., & Striegel-Moore, R. H. (1984). Women and weight: A normative discontent. In T. B. Sonderegger (Ed.), *Psychology and gender: Nebraska symposium on motivation* (Vol. 32, pp. 267–307). Lincoln: University of Nebraska Press.

Russell, G. F. M. (1979). Bulimia nervosa: An ominous variant of anorexia nervosa. *Psychological Medicine, 9,* 429–448.

Safer, D. L., Telch, C. F., & Agras, W. S. (2001). Dialectical behavior therapy for bulimia nervosa. *American Journal of Psychiatry, 158,* 632–634.

Schmidt, U., Lee, S., Beecham, J., Perkins, S., Treasure, J., Yi, I., et al. (2007). A randomized controlled trial of family therapy and cognitive behavior therapy guided self-care for adolescents with bulimia nervosa and related disorders. *American Journal of Psychiatry, 164,* 591–598.

Shafran, R., Lee, M., Payne, E., & Fairburn, C. G. (2007). An experimental analysis of body checking. *Behaviour Research and Therapy, 45,* 113–121.

Shapiro, J. R., Berkman, N. D., Brownley, K. A., Sedway, J. A., Lohr, K. N., & Bulik, C. M. (2007). Bulimia nervosa treatment: A systematic review of randomized controlled trials. *International Journal of Eating Disorders, 40,* 321–336.

Smyth, J. M., Heron, K. E., Sliwinski, M. J., Wonderlich, S. A., Crosby, R. D., Mitchell, J. E., et al. (2007). Daily and momentary mood and stress are associated with binge eating and vomiting in bulimia nervosa patients in the natural environment. *Journal of Consulting and Clinical Psychology, 75,* 629–638.

Somerville, K., & Cooper, M. (2007). Using imagery to identify and characterise core beliefs in women with bulimia nervosa, dieting and non-dieting women. *Eating Behaviors, 8,* 450–456.

Steinhausen, H. C., & Weber, S. (2009). The outcome of bulimia nervosa: Findings from one-quarter century of research. *American Journal of Psychiatry, 166,* 1331–1341.

Striegel-Moore, R., Leslie, D., Petrill, S. A., Garvin, V., & Rosenheck, R. A. (2000). One-year use and cost of inpatient and outpatient services among female and male patients with an eating disorder: Evidence from a national database of health insurance claims. *International Journal of Eating Disorders, 27,* 381–389.

Strober, M., Freeman, R., Lampert, C., Diamond, J., & Kaye, W. (2000). Controlled family study of anorexia nervosa and bulimia nervosa: Evidence of shared liability and transmission of partial syndromes. *American Journal of Psychiatry, 157,* 393–401.

Swami, V., Frederick, D. A., Aavik, T., Alcalay, L., Allik, J., Anderson, D., et al. (2010). The attractive female body weight and female body dissatisfaction in 26 countries across 10 world regions: Results of the International Body Project I. *Personality and Social Psychology Bulletin, 36,* 309–325.

Tanofsky-Kraff, M., & Wilfley, D. E. (2010). Interpersonal psychotherapy for bulimia nervosa and binge-eating disorder. In C. M. Grilo & J. E. Mitchell (Eds.), *The treatment of eating disorders: A clinical handbook* (pp. 271–293). New York: Guilford Press.

Thompson, M. P., & Light, L. S. (2011). Examining gender differences in risk factors for suicide attempts made 1 and 7 years later in a nationally representative sample. *Journal of Adolescent Health, 48,* 391–397.

Tozzi, F., Thornton, L. M., Klump, K. L., Fichter, M. M., Halmi, K. A., Kaplan, A. S., et al. (2005). Symptom fluctuation in eating disorders: Correlates of diagnostic crossover. *American Journal of Psychiatry, 162,* 732–740.

Wade, T. D. (2007). A retrospective comparison of purging type disorders: Eating disorder not otherwise specified and bulimia nervosa. *International Journal of Eating Disorders, 40,* 1–6.

Walsh, B. T., Sysko, R., & Parides, M. K. (2005). Early response to desipramine among women with bulimia nervosa. *International Journal of Eating Disorders, 39,* 72–75.

Walsh, B. T., Wilson, G. T., Loeb, K. L., Devlin, M. J., Pike, K. M., Roose, S. P., et al. (1997). Medication and psychotherapy in the treatment of bulimia nervosa. *American Journal of Psychiatry, 154,* 523–531.

Wegner, K. E., Smyth, J. M., Crosby, R. D., Wittrock, D., Wonderlich, S. A., & Mitchell, J. E. (2002). An evaluation of the relationship between binge eating in the natural environment using ecological momentary assessment. *International Journal of Eating Disorders, 32,* 352–361.

Wells, L. A., & Sadowski, C. A. (2001). Bulimia nervosa: An update and treatment recommendations. *Current Opinion in Pediatrics, 13,* 591–597.

Whittal, M. L., Agras, W. S., & Gould, R. (1999). Bulimia nervosa: A meta-analysis of psychosocial and pharmacological treatments. *Behavior Therapy, 30,* 117–135.

Wilfley, D. E., Agras, W. S., Telch, C. F., Rossiter, E. M., Schneider, J. A., Cole, A. G., et al. (1993). Group cognitive-behavioral and group interpersonal psychotherapy for the nonpurging bulimic individual: A controlled comparison. *Journal of Consulting and Clinical Psychology, 61,* 296–305.

Wilfley, D. E., Crow, S. J., Hudson, J. I., Mitchell, J. E., Berkowitz, R. I., Blakesley, V., et al. (2008). Efficacy of sibutramine for the treatment of binge eating disorder: A randomized multicenter placebo-controlled double-blind study. *American Journal of Psychiatry, 165,* 51–58.

Wilson, G. T., & Fairburn, C. G. (2002). Treatments for eating disorders. In P. E. Nathan & J. M. Gorman (Eds.), *A guide to treatments that work* (pp. 559–592). New York: Oxford University Press.

Wilson, G. T., Fairburn, C. G., & Agras, W. S. (1997). Cognitive-behavioral therapy for bulimia nervosa. In D. M. Garner & P. E. Garfinkel (Eds.), *Handbook of treatment for eating disorders* (2nd ed., pp. 67–93). New York: Guilford Press.

Wilson, G. T., Loeb, K. L., Walsh, B. T., Labouvie, E., Petkova, E., Liu, X., et al. (1999). Psychological versus pharmacological treatments of bulimia nervosa: Predictors and processes of change. *Journal of Consulting and Clinical Psychology, 67,* 451–459.

Wilson, R. R. (1996). *Don't panic: Taking control of anxiety attacks.* New York: HarperCollins.

Index